I0434355

Building a Healthy Lifestyle

Building a Healthy Lifestyle

A Simple Nutrition and Fitness Approach

Mary El-Baz

iUniverse, Inc.
New York Lincoln Shanghai

Building a Healthy Lifestyle
A Simple Nutrition and Fitness Approach

All Rights Reserved © 2004 by Mary El-Baz

No part of this book may be reproduced or transmitted in any form or by any means, graphic, electronic, or mechanical, including photocopying, recording, taping, or by any information storage retrieval system, without the written permission of the publisher.

iUniverse, Inc.

For information address:
iUniverse, Inc.
2021 Pine Lake Road, Suite 100
Lincoln, NE 68512
www.iuniverse.com

Please note that this book is to help you achieve a healthier lifestyle and is not intended to replace your health care provider. Ideas expressed in this book cannot be used to diagnose or treat individual health problems.

ISBN: 0-595-32506-8 (pbk)
ISBN: 0-595-66614-0 (cloth)

Printed in the United States of America

—*To my family and dearest friends who built and are enjoying healthier lifestyles*

Contents

Introduction

A healthy and fit body can be yours! It all begins with incremental changes that, gradually, make a big, beneficial healthful difference. Being knowledgeable about your body's nutritional needs for daily life allows you to make intelligent food choices that will maximize your health and well-being and minimize poor dietary habits, weight issues, and chronic health problems.

People today are living healthier lives. Lifestyle changes, public-health improvements, and improved health care have combined to extend longevity. Remarkable advances in medical science, technology, and nutrition are allowing us to have longer and healthier lives. Of these advances, bettering our nutrition is under our individual control. We can lead healthier lives by eating well. However, for some of us, our knowledge of basic nutrition and its effect on our daily lives stopped in grade school. We learned about the four basic food groups and about essential vitamins and minerals, and about the importance of physical activity. Now, as adults, so much of that knowledge has been buried beneath the stress of our hectic lives. We have families to raise, aging parents to care for, excessive job demands to meet, mortgages to pay, and long commutes to endure. The day ends and we cannot sleep. When do we find the time to exercise or de-stress or plan a healthy meal? Isn't there a quick fix to solve our low-energy needs? Can't we just take the latest antioxidant or anti-inflammatory dietary supplement that we've read about, and feel like new again?

It is not that simple. So, many of us begin feeling run-down; we feel drained by our lifestyle, and we decide to regain our health by eating better and exercising more. We rediscover the basics of good nutrition and its healing effect on our overall well-being. However, nutrition today is more scientific. More research is being done to help us understand how whole foods add to our well-being. We have more information at our fingertips—thanks to the Internet—to improve our health through the advances in nutritional research.

We have more information on diet's role in preventing age-related diseases, and some of that information is in terms the average person can understand.

This guide offers basic information to help you make intelligent choices in maintaining or improving your health. Nutrition biochemistry and medical terms have been translated into language you can understand. Many books written by doctors give detailed explanations of the biochemistry of nutrition and your body. If you want the medical explanation of how cholesterol is manufactured and used in your body or a description of metabolic byproducts on the atomic level and how they are detrimental to your health, or a discussion of the theory and study of what dietary supplements of vitamins, minerals, and herbal extracts you should take for optimum health, read books on those topics written by those who hold advanced degrees in those fields.

If you want a simple version of the principles of healthful nutrition and body fitness, this is the book for you. These principles are based on building and maintaining variety, balance and moderation in your diet, physical activity and mental outlook. We can begin our journey by looking at the old "healthful nutrition" adage:

- Be sure to eat a variety of foods, including plenty of vegetables, fruits, and whole-grain products.

- Include low-fat dairy products, lean meats, poultry, fish, and legumes.

- Drink lots of water and go easy on the salt, sugar, alcohol, and saturated fat.

- Include regular physical activity and stress management.

- Do not smoke.

- If you drink alcoholic beverages, do so in moderation.

It is important to understand how beneficial this advice really is. Finding out what this means, why you should follow these guidelines, and how to incorporate this information into your daily life in order to improve your nutritional, physical, and emotional health can be confusing. The hardest part of living healthier is getting started. This book gives you the simple guidelines to help you change your diet and become more active. Here's how to start:

- Learn about nutrition and the health benefits you reap from following good nutrition in Chapter 1, **The Stuff You're Made Of: Carbohydrates, Fats, Proteins, Fiber, and Water.**

- Understand the importance of antioxidants, anti-inflammatory nutrients, and vitamins and minerals in your health in Chapters 2 and 3, **Antioxidants** and **Vitamins and Minerals.**

- Make use of your new knowledge of healthy nutrition by following the eating plan outlined in Chapter 4, **A Reasonable Eating Plan.**

- Determine how your weight affects your health and easy ways to become more fit, from your muscles to your skin, in Chapter 5, **Body Fitness.**

- Discover simple, relaxing techniques that improve your sleep and overall health, both physical and emotional, in Chapter 6, **Relax; Take It Easy.**

- Build a healthy lifestyle and live it for the rest of your life, in Chapter 7, **Leading a Healthy Lifestyle for the Rest of Your Life.**

1

The Stuff You're Made Of: Carbohydrates, Fats, Protein, Fiber, and Water

Everyone should balance his or her intake of carbohydrates, fats, fiber, protein, and water during the day to reduce the risk of chronic disease while providing an adequate intake of essential nutrients. Well, how do you do that? What do you need to know? Let's briefly review the components of basic human nutrition.

Energy is required to sustain the body's various functions, including breathing, blood circulation, physical activity, and making protein. This energy is supplied by carbohydrates, fats, and protein in the diet. The energy that is released by these nutrients is measured in calories. Both carbohydrates and protein contain 4 calories per gram, whereas fat contains 9 calories per gram. Just by looking at these amounts, we can see that it takes more than twice the amount of energy to burn a gram of fat than it does to burn a gram of protein or carbohydrate.

The energy balance of a person depends on his or her dietary energy intake and energy utilization. The energy requirement to maintain this balance in a healthy adult depends on that person's age, gender, weight, height, and level of physical activity. The energy content of a food is determined by how much protein, carbohydrate, and fat it contains. If you don't use these nutrients immediately after you eat them, your body will store them in the form of body fat and put them away for use between meals and overnight. A simple rule to understand is that if you consume more than you use, you will gain weight. It doesn't matter if it is in the form of protein, carbohydrates, or fats.

The primary role of carbohydrates is to provide energy to cells in the body, particularly the brain, which is our only carbohydrate-dependent organ. Carbohydrates are the body's primary fuel source, because it is easier for the body to break down a gram of carbohydrate for energy than to break down a gram of fat. In order for your body to use fat as energy, you either have to be doing something aerobic (walking, running, biking, skating) for at least fifteen minutes, or be completely depleted of carbohydrates so your body has no other choice than to use stored body fat for energy.

Depleting the body of carbohydrates in order to force the body to use stored body fat for energy is the basis of many popular low-carbohydrate weight-loss plans. Reducing the amount of carbohydrates required by the body to a minimum level for a certain period, and eating more proteins and fat to make up for the calories not eaten as carbohydrates forces the body to use its fat stores for energy, causing weight loss. Once an individual reaches the desired weight, to stop weight loss and maintain the desired weight level, he or she adds carbohydrates back into the diet a few grams at a time, thus replacing some of the protein and fat being eaten for energy upkeep. The individual then eats this number of grams of carbohydrate foods per day, balancing caloric needs with protein and fat foods, for weight maintenance. To avoid vitamin and mineral deficiencies that may result from restricting the wide variety of plant food sources, the eating plan usually incorporates dietary supplements.

These types of eating plans create an imbalance of nutrients in the diet and deprive the body of its highest-quality energy source, reduce the efficiency of digestion and metabolism, make it harder for the body to replenish its required fat stores, and may encourage muscle tissue break down. As a temporary eating approach, these eating plans may not harm your health.

As a longer-term approach to well-being and health, however, you want to strive for a balance in your consumption of carbohydrates, proteins, and fats in order to give your body an energy balance that will allow you to feel your best and give you the energy, and then some, for your daily activities. Here are some guidelines for you to consider in planning your own lifelong healthy eating plan.

Most dietitians recommended that adults get 50 to 60 percent of their daily calories from carbohydrates, 30 percent from fat, and 10 to 20 percent from protein. Recently, a new report from the Institute of Medicine of the National

Academies (an organization that provides science-based advice on matters of biomedical science, medicine and health to the nation) is recommending that adults get 45 to 65 percent of their daily calories from carbohydrates, 20 to 35 percent from fat, and 10 to 35 percent from protein.[1]

In the United States, the Food and Drug Administration (FDA) helps us understand how to choose foods to follow these nutritional guidelines by requiring a Nutrition Facts label on food products and a footnote section of general dietary information of important nutrients on larger packages of food products. Find a food product in your pantry, and take a look at the Nutrition Facts panel to get a better idea of how the information on the label is organized. There's more about the information on the label in the Nutrition Facts panel in Chapter 4.

The footnote section helps you make intelligent food choices because it shows dietary advice; it is not about a specific food product. It shows the key nutrients that you should eat every day, depending on a 2,000- or 2,500-calorie diet. Those nutrients are total fat, saturated fat, cholesterol, potassium, total carbohydrate, dietary fiber, and protein. For a 2,000-calorie diet, total fat is listed as no more than 65 grams per day (g/day), total carbohydrate is listed as 300 g/day, dietary fiber is listed as 25 g/day, and protein is listed as 50 g/day.

Following the dietary guidelines for carbohydrate percentages (50 to 60% of daily calories), the body requires about 125 to 150 grams of carbohydrates a day for every 1,000 calories. That is, because 500 calories is 50 percent of 1,000 calories, and carbohydrates contain 4 calories per gram, hence 125 grams. Likewise, 600 calories (60% of 1,000 calories) divided by 4 calories per gram equals 150 grams. For fat percentages (30% of daily calories), the body requires about 33.33 grams. Because fat contains 9 calories per gram, 300 calories (30% of 1,000) divided by 9 calories per gram equals 33.33 grams. For protein percentages (10 to 20% of daily calories), the requirement is between 25 and 50 grams of protein per day. Because protein has 4 calories per gram, 100 calories (10% of 1,000 calories) divided by 4 calories per gram equals 25 grams and 200 calories (20% of 1,000 calories) divided by 4 calories per gram equals 50 grams.

---

1. *Dietary Reference Intakes for Energy, Carbohydrate, Fiber, Fat, Fatty Acids, Cholesterol, Protein, and Amino Acids (2002).* www.iom.edu. Copyright 2002 by the National Academies. All rights reserved.

Accordingly, on a diet of 2,000 calories a day, you should eat between 250 and 300 grams of carbohydrates, about 67 grams of fat, and between 25 and 50 grams of protein. So the nutrient listings in the footnote section of the Nutrition Facts panel for a 2,000-calorie diet for total carbohydrates of 300 g/day, total fats of 65 g/day, and protein of 50 g/day are the maximum amount of these nutrients you should be eating daily. This nutrient listing helps us calculate our daily nutritional needs and plan our meals for healthy eating.

Carbohydrates

Carbohydrates are composed of starches (complex carbohydrates) and sugars (simple carbohydrates). Complex carbohydrates take longer to digest and are usually packed with fiber, vitamins, and minerals. Examples are vegetables, breads, cereals, legumes, and pasta. Simple carbohydrates are digested quickly. Many simple carbohydrates contain refined sugars and a few essential vitamins and minerals. Examples include fruits, fruit juice, milk, yogurt, honey, molasses, maple syrup, and sugar. It used to be recommended that we limit our intake of simple carbohydrates and get most of our fuel requirements from the starches. Complex carbohydrates were thought to trigger smaller increases in blood glucose (blood sugar) than sugary foods. But researchers had found that the body's blood sugar or glycemic response to complex carbohydrates varies considerably. Recent research has changed this line of thought. Now, the basic indicator of how blood glucose responds to dietary carbohydrates is the *glycemic index*.

Glycemic Index of Carbohydrate Foods

The glycemic index ranks carbohydrate foods according to how quickly they release glucose into your bloodstream. Foods that are at the higher end of the glycemic index break down quickly during digestion, causing rapid blood sugar changes that can affect your mood and desire to eat again. Foods that are on the lower end of the glycemic index usually break down more slowly, releasing glucose gradually into the bloodstream, thus maintaining a stable blood sugar level over a longer period.

There are many books available written by physicians that explain the biochemistry of your body's delicate glucose and insulin balance, and what can happen when an imbalance occurs. They discuss type 2 diabetes, insulin resistance, and Syndrome X, all medical conditions related to an imbalance in blood sugar and insulin levels. The point of this book is to introduce you to foods that help maintain the balance between glucose and insulin in your body, so that you will have the energy you need for your daily activities, and those sometimes strenuous activities, and for overall good health.

The level of blood sugar in our blood is one mechanism that controls hunger. When your blood glucose level falls below normal, you feel hungry. When you eat, and as your food is digested, carbohydrates in the food are converted into glucose and enter your bloodstream. As your blood sugar rises, your pancreas secretes insulin to clean up the excess blood sugar. This process repeats as your blood glucose levels fall below normal.

High-glycemic foods can cause us to be hungrier more often, thus we overeat (ingesting more calories than our bodies can use), which leads to obesity. Here's what happens when you eat a high-glycemic food or meal. There is a rapid rise in your blood sugar level. This overstimulates the pancreas to release a much larger amount of insulin. This large amount of insulin rapidly cleans up the excess sugar in your bloodstream, causing the blood sugar level to dip quickly below normal. Now you're hungry again! So you eat once more after you have just eaten! This process can lead to overeating and weight gain. Eating low-glycemic foods helps slow down this cycle by delaying the return of hunger. As a result, meals are spaced further apart, increasing the satiety of foods eaten, sustaining more energy, maintaining stable blood sugar levels, and reducing calorie intake. This, ultimately, is weight control.

Low-glycemic eating plans focus on reducing the intake of foods that elevate insulin and stimulate fat storage. Non-carbohydrate foods, such as protein and fats, do not raise your blood sugar much, if at all. Low-glycemic foods can be mixed with modest quantities of high-glycemic foods without losing their hunger-reducing effect. Keeping the higher-glycemic foods to a minimum and eating them in combination with low-glycemic foods will not significantly elevate insulin levels. Just make sure that the foods you choose have a significant amount of soluble fiber! That is fiber that slows digestion, which reduces the glycemic effect. Also, even though low-glycemic foods do not stimulate fat storage as efficiently as high-glycemic foods, they still contain calories. Serving and portion sizes do matter.

A chart of the glycemic index of foods is not included. Why? The glycemic index ranks only individual foods, not meal combinations. This does not give you any idea of the blood sugar effects after a meal. The glycemic index does not account for portion size or calories, and both are very important in maintaining weight control. Rather than listing foods by their glycemic index rating, we list foods that are preferred in more quantities than others.

A good understanding of high- and low-carbohydrate foods and their effect on your body will help you make better food choices for health and well-being. Eating a wide variety of fiber-rich foods (such as vegetables, fruits, whole grains), along with small amounts of healthy fats (such as nuts and olive oil), daily is the best way to control your weight and blood sugar, vitamins and minerals. In effect, you are reducing saturated fat (the major source is fast foods), reducing refined sugar (soft drinks are a major source), and increasing fiber in your diet by reducing refined foods.

Carbohydrates Recap

Increase your intake of low-carbohydrate (slow-acting carbohydrates) foods, which are slowly digested and absorbed to help maintain blood sugar levels. Slow-acting carbohydrates include:

- Most vegetables, such as cooked and salad greens, the cabbage (cruciferous) family of vegetables
- Most fruit, such as berries, apples, pears, oranges, grapes, cherries, grapefruit, peaches, plums, kiwi fruit, and firm bananas
- Dried peas and beans, such as lentils, lima beans, kidney beans, haricot beans, chickpeas, and baked beans
- Whole grains and whole-grain cereals, such as barley, buckwheat, bulgur, rolled oats, barley bran, rice bran, and oat bran
- Heavy whole-grain breads, such as pumpernickel
- Basmati rice
- Pasta

Moderate your intake of high-carbohydrate (quick-acting carbohydrates) foods. Quick-acting carbohydrates include:

- Vegetables such as corn, white and sweet potatoes, yams, green peas, beets, carrots, parsnips, rutabaga, pumpkin
- Fruits such as watermelon, overripe bananas, cantaloupe, honeydew melon, pineapple, mango, guava, papaya, dried fruits

- Refined bread and bakery products, dessert products, candy, soft drinks

Dietary Fiber

Dietary fiber is actually considered a carbohydrate, the non-digestible carbohydrates from plants that we eat. These fibers are too complex for our bodies to break down. The plant cell wall structure of the nutrient remains intact during the digestive process. There are two types of fiber: *soluble* or *viscous,* and *insoluble* or *fermentable.*

Soluble or viscous fiber slows digestion of foods from the stomach to the small intestine, which results in a sensation of fullness. This delayed effect results in a slow and steady release of glucose (blood sugar) from accompanying carbohydrates. Soluble fiber binds with bile acids and cholesterol, interfering with the absorption of dietary fat and cholesterol, as well as with the recirculation of cholesterol and bile acids, resulting in reduced blood cholesterol levels.

Insoluble or fermentable fiber assists in regulating normal gastrointestinal functioning and in keeping the colon clean. Fermentable fibers also help maintain healthy populations of friendly bacteria in the large intestine, where this type of fiber is fermented. These bacteria play an important role in the immune system by preventing disease-causing bacteria from surviving in the intestinal tract. As is the case with insoluble fiber, fibers that are not fermentable in the large intestine help maintain bowel regularity by speeding up the time it takes food to pass through the large intestines, thereby diluting toxic and carcinogenic compounds. Bowel regularity is associated with a decreased risk for colon cancer and hemorrhoids.

To keep that healthful balance of friendly bacteria, besides adding fermentable fiber to your diet, be sure to eat on a regular basis yogurt, acidophilus milk, kefir, and other cultured milk products (look for the statement "live cultures" on all these products' labels), and fermented foods such as miso, raw sauerkraut, raw pickles, and pickled Korean cabbage (kim chee) that have not been pasteurized. These foods, called probiotics, contain friendly bacteria strains that are in your digestive tract: acidophilus, bifidus, and lactobacillus. Dietary supplements containing these bacteria are available. These are especially handy in maintaining digestive health when you are traveling abroad. Also, if you are taking antibiotics, it is a good idea to eat probiotic foods to replenish the friendly bacteria that has been killed along with the bad bacteria.

So, your grandma was right when she told you, "Spinach is the broom of the stomach, but sauerkraut is the vacuum cleaner!"

Insoluble fibers can be found in foods such as wheat bran, whole grains and whole-grain cereals, nuts, seeds, fruits and vegetables (particularly turnip greens, mustard greens, collard greens, chard, broccoli, cauliflower, cabbage, Brussels sprouts, green beans, split peas, lentils, lima beans, carrots, cucumbers, celery, zucchini, and tomatoes). Soluble fiber is found in the pectin in fruits (particularly apples, pears, strawberries, and blueberries), vegetables (artichokes, legumes), seeds, oatmeal, and oat bran. You should always drink water when eating fiber to prevent constipation, especially when taking it in supplement form or eating low-moisture foods, such as whole grains and nuts. Changing from a low-fiber to a high-fiber intake should be done in increments to avoid gastrointestinal distress such as bloating and gas. Sources of insoluble fiber include whole grains such as bran.

The recommended adequate intake (AI) for total fiber is set at 38 g/day for adult men under 50 and 25 g/day for adult women under 50. For adults 50 and older, the total fiber recommendation is 30 g/day for men and 21 g/day for women, because of their decreased food consumption. Unfortunately, most of us are getting from 10 to 15 grams of dietary fiber a day. Dietary fiber is listed on the Nutrition Facts food label. It does not separate the fiber into insoluble and soluble. Use this information as a guide in selecting foods high in fiber when you are planning your meals.

Fats

Fat is a major source of energy for the body and aids in the absorption of fat-soluble vitamins and other food components. The amount of fat that can be eaten can vary greatly while still meeting daily energy needs. Fats in our diet promote healthy cell membranes. Cells without a healthy membrane lose their ability to hold water and vital nutrients. Because cell membranes are made up of fat, the integrity and fluidity of our cell membranes is determined in large part by the type of fat we eat.

There are saturated, cholesterol, monounsaturated, and polyunsaturated fats, and hydrogenated or trans fats.

- **Saturated fats:** These fats are solid at room temperature. They are found in animal foods, such as butter, lard, and coconut and palm oil. Cholesterol is a form of saturated fat and is found in liver and eggs. To some degree, the body produces saturated fat and cholesterol.

- **Trans fats (trans fatty acids) or hydrogenated and partially hydrogenated fats:** This fat is a manufactured fat created by adding hydrogen molecules to liquid vegetable oil and is semi-solid at room temperature. Margarine and vegetable shortening are hydrogenated fats.

- **Polyunsaturated and monounsaturated fats:** These are vegetable oils and are liquid at room temperature. Polyunsaturated oil contains omega-6 (linoleic acid) essential fatty acids (EFA). Omega-6 is found in high concentrations in corn, soybean, safflower, cottonseed, and sunflower oil. Monounsaturated oil (such as olive oil, canola oil, peanut oil, and in avocados and nuts) contains omega-9 (oleic acid) fatty acids. The body also produces some monounsaturated fat. Omega-3 (linolenic acid or alpha-linolenic acid) essential fatty acids are found in flaxseed oil, walnuts, cold-water fish (salmon, tuna, sardines, halibut, and herring), special eggs from chickens fed a vegetarian diet, and greens such as kale and purslane. These cold-water fish and their oils also contain DHA (docosahexaenoic acid) fatty acids, which is a part of the omega-3 fatty acids family. DHA is the main structural component of brain cells. There is increasing evidence that DHA is essential for mental functioning throughout your life. If your mother ever told you that fish is "brain food," she's right.

Researchers believe that diets containing large amounts of saturated or hydrogenated fats produce cell membranes that are hard and lack fluidity. On the other hand, diets rich in omega-3 fats produce cell membranes with a high degree of fluidity. A growing body of scientific research indicates that these healthy fats or essential fatty acids help prevent a wide range of medical problems, including cardiovascular disease, depression, asthma, and rheumatoid arthritis. Essential fatty acids are grouped into two families: omega-6 and the omega-3 essential fatty acids. Omega-6 fatty acids promote inflammation, blood clotting, and tumor growth, while omega-3 fatty acids work in just the opposite manner.

Foods rich in omega-6 fatty acids are generally baked, fried in vegetable oils, and processed. Because of our modern diets, we ingest a high proportion of foods rich in these fatty acids, which increase our bodies' production of the pro-inflammatory hormone-like substance called prostaglandins. To regain our health and lead an anti-inflammatory lifestyle, we must rebalance the body's ratio of omega-3 fatty acids to the omega-6 fatty acids.

The Food and Nutrition Board of the Institute of Medicine recommends that people consume at least 2 percent of their total daily calories as omega-3 fats. Since our bodies synthesize saturated fat and cholesterol and they have no known beneficial role in preventing chronic diseases, they are not required in our diets and no Adequate Intake (AI) requirements have been set for them. The recommended AI for omega-6 fatty acid is 17 g/day for men and 12 g/day for women. The recommended AI for omega-3 fatty acid is 1.6 g/day for men and 1.1 g/day for women. To meet this recommendation, a person eating 2,000 calories per day should eat at least 4 grams of omega-3 fats. This goal can be easily met by adding just two foods to your diet: flaxseeds and wild-caught salmon. Two tablespoons of flaxseeds contain 3.5 grams of omega-3 fats, while a 4-ounce piece of salmon contains 1.5 grams of omega-3 fats.

Total Fat is listed on the Nutrition Facts food label as well. Total Fat may be separated into amounts of Saturated (Sat), Trans, Polyunsaturated, and Monounsaturated Fat that add up to the total fat in the food product. Use this information as a guide in selecting foods with fat when you are planning your meals. Sources of total fat are butter, margarine, vegetable oils, whole milk, visible fat on meat and poultry, invisible fat in fish, shellfish, some plant products such as seeds and nuts, and bakery products.

Guidelines on Fat Consumption

- **Reduce the Amount of Saturated Fat and Avoid Trans Fat:** The more saturated fat you eat, the more cholesterol your body produces. This builds up in your blood and can increase the risks of your developing heart disease and other health problems. The problem with trans fat is that the body cannot break them down and use them as it uses other fatty acids. Trans fatty acids are stiff and can build up in the body. The areas affected include the lining of blood vessels and brain surfaces, where the buildup can cause dysfunction. Trans fatty acids are linked to increased inflammation, poor immunity, obesity, heart disease, diabetes, high cholesterol, and acceleration of the aging process.

  It is hard to avoid trans fatty acids in the typical American diet. Partially hydrogenated oil is often an ingredient in processed foods, and fast-foods and cheaper foods tend to include these fats because they stabilize the other ingredients. Read the Nutrition Facts label on packaged goods and on lists of ingredients. The best advice is to avoid processed and prepackaged foods and fried foods from fast-food places and restaurants.

- **Use More Olive Oil:** The oleic acid in olive oil helps the body produce cell membranes with a high degree of fluidity. The body uses the monounsaturated fats in olive oil to produce substances that are relatively anti-inflammatory. By reducing inflammation, these fats can help reduce the severity of arthritis symptoms. It is believed that the vitamin E in olive oil also protects cells from cellular damage. Olive oil also contains plant substances called polyphenols, which are powerful antioxidants. One of the polyphenols found in olives is thought to act as an anti-inflammatory. The most effective type of olive oil from a health standpoint is the "extra-virgin" variety. Extra-virgin olive oil contains the highest density of polyphenols. So, olive oil has both antioxidant and anti-inflammatory properties, giving you more bang for your buck, so to speak!

  Use olive oil regularly in your cooking, eat more olives, or add one or two tablespoons a day to your diet. Monounsaturated oils should be stored in a cool, dark place. Although refrigeration can cause olive oil to thicken and darken, bringing it to room temperature will restore its color and fluidity. Prolonged storage at room temperature will cause olive oil to lose its taste and protective qualities.

- **Limit the Use of Polyunsaturated Oils and Avoid Rancid Fats:** Polyunsaturated oils, including the omega-3 fats, are extremely susceptible to damage from heat, light, and oxygen. Omega-3 oils, in particular, should never be heated but only used as a dressing. When exposed to heat, light, or oxygen for too long, the fatty acids in the oil become oxidized, a scientific term that simply means that the oil becomes rancid. Rancidity not only alters the oil's flavor and smell, it also diminishes the nutritional value. Oxidized oils promote inflammation, cancer, arthritis, cardiovascular disease, and premature aging of cells and tissues.

  Learn to identify rancid fat with your nose. You can do this by allowing cooking oil to sit out for a few days. Rancid oil has a linseed-oil type of smell (linseed oil is oxidized flaxseed oil). If you smell the same odor in nuts, chips, flour, or baked goods, throw them away. Under most circumstances, the problem of rancidity only arises when the oils are removed from their natural food package. For example, the hard shell of the flaxseed protects the oil inside the seed from heat, light, and oxygen. Flaxseeds also contain antioxidant compounds, such as vitamin E, that provide additional protection against oxidation. But when the seed is pressed to isolate the oil, the oil becomes vulnerable to the elements.

Store oils rich in polyunsaturated fatty acids in tightly closed, dark glass containers in the refrigerator.

- **Hiccup!** Sometimes fat in your diet may cause indigestion. To aid digestion, add bitters to your diet. Europeans have taken them before meals to aid digestion for more than 2,000 years. Bitter herbs such as gentian, dandelion root, and globe artichoke stimulate the stomach's production of digestive fluids. These digestive fluids help your body absorb the nutrients from your food. Bitter foods like tart red grape juice, arugula, watercress, and dandelion greens also work when you incorporate them into meals.

  You can buy bitters in supermarkets (the liquor section) or in natural food stores. Angostura Bitters and Peychaud's Bitters are two common brands in the United States. A recommended amount is one teaspoonful of herbal bitters mixed in water about fifteen minutes before meals. Now you know why Italians drink those bitter aperitifs such as Campari, Aperol, or Cynar.

Proteins

Proteins form the major structural components of all the cells of the body. Along with amino acids, they function as enzymes, membrane carriers, and hormones. The Recommended Dietary Allowance (RDA) for both men and women is 0.8 grams per kilogram of body weight per day or 0.8 grams for every 2.2 pounds of body weight per day. Amino acids are the dietary components of protein. Protein is made up of twenty amino acids, eleven that the body can produce and nine that it cannot. These nine are called the essential amino acids and must be provided from dietary sources. All twenty amino acids must be present in your body at the same time to form protein.

Food sources that provide protein with the nine essential amino acids are animal proteins, such as meat, poultry, fish, eggs, milk, cheese, and yogurt. These types of proteins are called *complete proteins*. Proteins from plants, legumes, grains, seeds, and vegetables tend to be lacking in one or more of the essential amino acids. They are called *incomplete proteins*. Persons following a non-meat, non-dairy, non-egg, all-vegetable diet (vegan diet) usually eat combinations of sources of incomplete proteins to create the complete protein required.

Concerns about Mercury Levels in Fish

Nearly all fish and shellfish contain traces of mercury; therefore, people can be exposed to trace levels of methylmercury by eating fish. Mercury is an element and a metal. It finds its way into the food chain when naturally occurring mercury (such as from underwater volcanoes) or mercury from air pollutants is deposited into rivers and lakes. Once in the water, bacteria transform the airborne mercury into methylmercury. Larger, predatory species of fish, such as sharks and swordfish, absorb methylmercury from the water and ingest it when eating algae and smaller species of fish. We are also exposed to mercury through dental fillings known as dental amalgams.

There is some concern because methylmercury can accumulate in your bloodstream over time. Methylmercury is removed from the body naturally, but it may take over a year for the levels to drop significantly. While most people's fish consumption does not cause a health concern, high levels of mercury in the bloodstream can have an effect on the developing nervous systems of young children and unborn babies.

Therefore, the Food and Drug Administration (FDA) and the Environmental Protection Agency (EPA) (as of the writing of this book) have an advisory for women who may become pregnant, pregnant women, nursing mothers, and young children:

- Do not eat shark, swordfish, king mackerel, or tilefish because they contain high levels of mercury.

- Eat up to 12 ounces (two average meals) a week of a variety of fish and shellfish that are lower in mercury.

  - Five of the most commonly eaten fish that are low in mercury are shrimp, canned light tuna, salmon, pollock, and catfish.

  - Another commonly eaten fish, albacore tuna, has more mercury than canned light tuna. So, when choosing your two meals of fish and shellfish, you may eat up to 6 ounces (one average meal) of albacore tuna per week.

- Check local advisories about the safety of fish caught by family and friends in your local lakes, rivers, and coastal areas. If no advice is available, eat up to 6 ounces (one average meal) per week of fish you catch from local waters, but don't consume any other fish during that week.

Even though this advisory is for women of childbearing age and young children, those of us who are concerned about potential higher levels of mercury would be wise to follow the advisory as well.

Water

Water is indispensable and abundant in the body. It actually forms the major part of every tissue within the body and provides the medium for which most of the body's activities are conducted. Your body is approximately 70 percent fluid. This fluid helps your body maintain its temperature, metabolize fat, lubricate and cushion internal organs, transport nutrients, and flush out toxins. Drinking plenty of water helps maintain this fluid level, maximizes metabolic functioning, and flushes the resulting waste products out of your body. Your body excretes water constantly through sweat, urine, and exhaled air, which is why it's so important to replenish your body with an ample amount of water every day. Most health professionals agree that the average human body requires from eight to ten glasses of water a day. You obviously don't have to drink that much water each day because there is water in some of the foods we eat.

A simple calculation for determining your actual water requirements is to multiply your body weight by 0.6 and then divide it by 12. This will give you the number of 8-ounce glasses of water you need per day. For example, if you weigh 140 pounds, then 140 multiplied by 0.6 and the total divided by 12 equals seven 8-ounce glasses of water a day. If you weigh 200 pounds, then the calculation would determine that you would need ten 8-ounce glasses of water a day. Without feeling overwhelmed by quantity, you can reach this amount by drinking around 6 ounces of water about every two hours throughout the day.

If you are not drinking enough water, you may experience some symptoms of dehydration, such as fatigue, headaches, dry mouth and lips, thirst, dry skin, and confusion. When the body gets dehydrated, the body seeks water from other sources, including fat cells. If your fat cells have less water, there's less mobilization of fat for energy. You can also become dehydrated from vomiting, diarrhea, over-exposure to the sun, fever, diuretics, and natural diuretics such as alcohol and caffeine.

Several factors may increase your need for more water, depending on your weight. These factors include:

- Moderate exercise

- Consumption of at least one caffeinated beverage a day

- Consumption of at least one alcoholic beverage a day

- Air travel

- Travel to a different climate (hot to cold, cold to hot)

- A fever, cold, flu, or a minor illness

- A weight-loss program

For example, if you weigh between 110 and 140 pounds, increase your water intake by at least one glass daily. If you weigh between 140 and 175 pounds, increase your water intake by at least two glasses daily. If you weigh between 175 and 200 pounds, increase your water intake by at least three glasses daily.

Consider Filtered or Bottled Water

Depending on your community's public water system, you may want to install a household water filtration system for your drinking water. This can be a simple water-pitcher carbon filtration unit or dispenser, or a more complex filtration system attached to your water supply line. These systems don't purify the water; they just filter out some common contaminants, such as lead, copper, mercury, cadmium, benzene, toluene, trichloroethylene, chlorine, zinc, and sediments. Lead and copper appear due to the corrosion of household plumbing systems and the erosion of natural deposits. Mercury can appear due to the erosion of natural deposits and from runoff from landfills and cropland. Cadmium can appear due to corrosion of galvanized pipes and from runoff from waste batteries and paints. Benzene can appear due to discharge from factories and from leaching from gas storage tanks and landfills. Potential health effects from these contaminants can range from gastrointestinal distress and anemia to kidney, liver damage, and increased risk of cancer. You may want to have your water supply tested to determine your actual water treatment needs before you purchase a water treatment unit.

You may also decide to drink bottled water. Be aware that some leaching of plastic contaminants may be present in the water. Read the labels to determine what type of water treatment the bottled water has undergone. All spring water is not necessarily contaminant-free.

2

Antioxidants

Antioxidants are vitamins, minerals and enzymes that work on the cellular level and that function as cell protectors in our bodies. Antioxidants protect our bodies in the following manner: During normal cellular metabolism, oxygen, an essential element for life, can create damaging byproducts. These oxidized cellular byproducts, called free radicals, are highly unstable and steal components from other cellular molecules, such as fat, protein, or DNA, thereby spreading the damage. This damage continues in a chain reaction, and entire cells soon become damaged and die. This process, known as peroxidation, is helpful because it helps the body destroy cells that have outlived their usefulness and neutralizes viruses, bacteria, and parasites. However, when left unchecked, peroxidation also destroys or damages healthy cells.

Free radicals are also created by exposure to various environmental factors, such as pollution, tobacco smoke, radiation, and pesticides. Normally, the body can handle free radicals, but if antioxidants are unavailable, or if the free-radical production becomes excessive, damage can occur. Too many free radicals in our bodies may cause heart damage, cancer, cataracts, and a weak immune system leading to an increased risk of infections. Additionally, free radical damage accumulates with age.

Antioxidants bind to the free radicals and either transform them into non-damaging compounds or repair cellular damage. More important, antioxidants return to the surface of the cell to stabilize rather than damage other cellular components. Common vitamin antioxidants include vitamin C, and vitamin E in conjunction with the mineral selenium.

Phytochemicals are substances in plants that are being investigated for their antioxidant and anticancer activity and health-promoting potential. The phytochemicals called carotenoids (such as lutein, beta-carotene, and lycopene) have been shown to have powerful antioxidant properties. Another common phytochemical compound that may be familiar to you is soy isoflavones. Researchers are discovering more health benefits from these plant substances every year.

Here are some good food sources of common antioxidants and phytochemicals:

- **Vitamin C:** Also called ascorbic acid, vitamin C is a water-soluble (not stored in the body) vitamin found in all body fluids. It protects tissues from breakdown by free radical formation. Important sources include green leafy vegetables, broccoli, green peppers, tomatoes, raw cabbage, citrus fruits, strawberries, and potatoes.

- **Vitamin E:** A fat-soluble vitamin that can be stored with fat in the liver and other tissues. It decreases free radical damage in connective and organ tissue, accelerating wound healing and protecting tissue from damage. Vitamin E increases immunity and protects against cataracts and macular degeneration. Vitamin E protects cells from the cancerous effects of X-rays, chemicals, air pollutants, and ultraviolet light. Important sources include vegetable oil, nuts, seeds, whole grains, wheat germ, olives, avocados, green leafy vegetables, and fish-liver oil.

- **Carotenoids:** These potent phytochemicals are the fat-soluble pigments abundant in yellow, orange, red, and green fruits and vegetables. Beta-carotene, alpha-carotene, and beta-cryptoxanthin are carotenes that are converted into vitamin A (a vitamin essential for normal metabolism and health) or retinol (the active form of vitamin A) in the body.

  The provitamin-A carotenoid receiving the most research attention is beta-carotene. Special controls in our body limit how much beta-carotene becomes vitamin A, leaving the remainder to act as an antioxidant. It can disarm reactive oxygen molecules generated by sunlight and air pollution and prevent free radical damage to skin, eyes, and lungs. Beta-carotene is the most widely studied carotenoid. Evidence now strongly suggests that when taken as a separate supplement, it can have harmful effects.[1,2] Carrots, squash, broccoli, sweet potatoes, tomatoes, kale, collards, cantaloupe, peaches, and apricots are particularly rich sources of beta-carotene.

The carotenoid lycopene is responsible for the red color in fruits and vegetables, including tomatoes, red grapes, watermelon, and pink grape-fruit. It is also found in papayas and apricots. It does not convert to vitamin A but may have important cancer-fighting properties and other health benefits. The beneficial actions of most carotenes such as those in tomatoes, corn, and carrots appear to be enhanced by cooking them, especially in oil (preferably olive, canola, or another monounsaturated oil). Cooking increases their nutritional value by breaking down the tough cell walls and releasing the nutrients. For example, the body cannot obtain lycopene from raw tomatoes. The body best absorbs lycopene from cooked tomatoes (such as tomato juice and tomato sauce) along with a bit of dietary fat.

- **Selenium:** This mineral is thought to help fight cell damage by oxygen-derived compounds and thus may help protect against cancer. It works together with vitamin E. It is best to get selenium through foods, because large doses of the supplement form can be toxic. Good food sources include fish, shellfish, red meat, whole grains, Brazil nuts, eggs, chicken, and garlic.

- **Green Tea:** Green tea is the unfermented leaf of the tea plant, *Camellia sinensis*, which contains the phytochemicals known as catechins. Catechins lower cholesterol, improve fat metabolism, and have significant anticancer and antibacterial effects.

- **Flavonoids:** The phytochemicals known as flavonoids are the largest group of several thousand compounds belonging to the antioxidant-rich polyphenol family. Laboratory studies have shown that specific flavonoids suppress tumor growth, prevent blood clots, and have anti-inflammatory properties.

1. The Alpha-Tocopherol, Beta Carotene Cancer Prevention Study Group. The effects of vitamin E and beta carotene on the incidence of lung cancer and other cancers in male smokers. *New England Journal of Medicine* 1994;330:1029–35.
2. Omenn, G.S., Goodman, G., Thomquist, M., et al. The beta-carotene and retinol efficacy trial (CARET) for chemoprevention of lung cancer in high risk populations: smokers and asbestos-exposed workers. *Cancer Res* 1994;54(7 Suppl):2038s–43s

In general, flavonoids are found in celery, cranberries, onions, kale, dark chocolate, broccoli, apples, cherries, berries, tea, red wine or purple grape juice, parsley, soybeans, tomatoes, eggplant, and thyme. Other important flavonoids are resveratrol, quercetin, and catechin. Resveratrol (found in red wine, grapes, olive oil) is a moderate antioxidant, not as potent as quercetin (citrus, apples, onions, black tea) or catechin (green teas).

- **Soy Isoflavones:** Soy (soybeans, veggie burgers, tempeh, tofu, soy milk) is full of high-quality protein and phytochemicals. It is rich in hormone-like compounds called isoflavones (genistein, daidzein, and biochanin A) that are similar to the hormones provided by the body. Isoflavones found in soy normalize hormone levels in the body and have been shown to stop the growth of hormone-dependent cancers.

- **Alpha Lipoic Acid:** Alpha lipoic acid (ALA) or lipoic acid is a natural antioxidant substance that is found in every cell of our bodies. It can be found in foods such as organ meats, vegetables (such as spinach, broccoli, Brussels sprouts, tomatoes, and peas), rice bran, and egg yolks. ALA is both water- and fat-soluble, enabling it to work both on the surface of cells and within them. Studies indicate that alpha lipoic acid supplements hold promise for treating various disorders, premature signs of aging, cancer prevention, liver ailments, diabetes, eye health, and skin health. In addition to its ability to protect cells from free radical damage, it enhances the effectiveness of the antioxidant vitamins C and E. These properties of lipoic acid may also benefit skin cells by improving skin texture. Many antioxidant skin care products are incorporating ALA into their formulations.

This potent and versatile antioxidant may someday be seen as a very important supplement. Research has determined that it is created in the human body and therefore is not an essential nutrient. For this reason, deficiencies of alpha lipoic acid are not known to occur in humans. There is no established recommended dietary allowance or adequate intake. The amount of alpha lipoic acid recommended by some doctors for general antioxidant protection is 100 mg, taken twice daily, although there is no clear evidence that such general use has any benefit. Alpha lipoic acid supplements may affect the optimal dose of medications used to control blood glucose in diabetics. Consult your doctor for guidance.

Other phytochemical compounds that you may have read about and their food sources include:

- Onions, garlic, leeks, and chives contain allyl sulfides, which reduce the risk of certain types of cancers and lower cholesterol and blood pressure.

- Turmeric contains curcumin, which has anti-inflammatory properties.

- Green leafy vegetables contain glutathione, which acts as an antioxidant.

- Broccoli, cauliflower, cabbage, Brussels sprouts, and bok choy contain indoles and isothiocyanates (sulforaphane), which reduce the risk of certain types of cancer.

- Seeds such as flaxseeds and sunflower seeds contain lignans, which have anti-inflammatory properties.

- Citrus fruit peels, cherries, and nuts contain monoterpenes, which act as antioxidants.

- Whole grains and legumes contain phytic acid, which acts as an antioxidant.

- Beans and legumes contain saponins, which reduce the risk of heart disease and cancer.

Antioxidants with Potent Anti-Inflammatory Properties

Inflammation is a natural reaction to injury or infection. It is a crucial aspect of the body's healing mechanism. Short-term inflammation can help the body heal from these injuries or infections, but if it persists too long or is in an area where it is not needed, it becomes chronic, prolonged, abnormal, or misplaced inflammation. It may result from food sensitivities that cause allergic-inflammatory responses or from a deficiency in essential fats and a variety of vitamins and minerals. Current medical views hold that this chronic inflammation may be the underlying cause of age-related diseases, such as heart disease and arthritis.

The discovery that certain natural substances produce marked anti-inflammatory effects on systemic inflammation has helped in the management of pain relief for some of these diseases. Recent studies have highlighted the anti-inflammatory benefits of some common foods: flaxseeds, ginger, and tur-meric.

- **Flaxseeds:** Flaxseeds are a rich source of omega-3 alpha-linolenic acid. Because our bodies are unable to produce omega-3 fatty acids, we must get them through our diet. Essential fatty acids protect us from the effects of high blood pressure, sticky platelets, inflammation, water retention, and lowered immune function. Numerous studies have shown that omega-3 fatty acids help lower cholesterol and prevent clotted arteries that may result in strokes, heart attacks, and thromboses. Scientists also think that omega-3 fatty acids have a beneficial role in other disease prevention, including hypertension, cancer, and inflammatory and immune disorders such as rheumatoid arthritis. Flaxseeds also contain lignans, which are phytochemicals known as phytoestrogens, compounds that have some estrogenic activity that may be helpful for post-menopausal women. Lignans also have antiviral, antibacterial, and antioxidant properties, but their anticancer effects have received the most research attention lately.

- **Ginger:** Ginger (*Zingiber officinale)* is known as a digestive aid and is a rhizome that contains enzymes and antioxidants. Ginger improves the digestion of proteins, is an effective treatment for nausea and motion sickness (for example, ginger ale), and strengthens the lining of the stomach. The polyphenols known as gingerols in fresh ginger have anti-inflammatory benefits and anticancer effects. When ginger is dried, its phytochemicals change to the more potent shogaols. These polyphenols have more powerful anti-inflammatory and analgesic effects. It is available as a fresh herb, in tablet, capsule, powdered, and liquid forms.

  An easy way to add ginger to your diet is to make fresh gingerroot tea. Take a small piece of gingerroot, peel and grate ½ teaspoon, grating lengthwise on the large holes of a grater. Put it into a small pot, pour in a cup of boiling water, let it steep for ten to fifteen minutes, and then strain it. You can add a sweetener of your choice and drink it hot or iced.

- **Turmeric:** Turmeric (*Curcuma longa)* is a member of the ginger family and is also a rhizome. It is best known as a spice in Indian curry. The volatile oil found in turmeric has shown significant anti-inflammatory activity in a variety of experiments. Its effective anti-inflammatory properties have made it a favorite among arthritis sufferers. Even more potent than its volatile oil is the yellow or orange pigment of turmeric, which is called curcumin. Curcumin is turmeric's active ingredient and is thought to have antioxidant and anti-inflammatory properties. Turmeric can be incorporated into the diet as a way to promote health. Used as a culinary spice, it can be eaten regularly and liberally. As a powder, it can be prepared as a tea. Curcumin is also available in tablets and capsules.

To make the tea, place ½ teaspoon of powder in a small pot, pour in a cup of boiling water, leave it to infuse for five minutes, and then strain it. You can add ginger or cardamom for more flavor. Drink one or two cups between meals.

Antioxidant and Anti-Inflammatory Recap

- Eat a large variety of deeply, brightly colored vegetables and fruits.

- Eat nuts, seeds, and olives more often.

- Use olive oil, canola oil, or various nut oils.

- Include more omega-3 fatty acids, such as cold-water, oily fish, or flaxseed oil or meal.

- Use ginger and turmeric more often.

- Eat more soy.

- Drink green tea.

- Select and eat berries as your main fruit.

- Eat dark chocolate (on occasion).

- Drink some red wine with a meal (on occasion).

- Limit the amount of saturated fats in your diet.

- Avoid sources of trans fatty acids, such as margarine and everything containing partially hydrogenated fat (vegetable shortening). They are linked to inflammation.

- Avoid polyunsaturated vegetable oils, such as corn or safflower oil. Their omega-6 fatty acids tend to promote inflammation.

3

Vitamins and Minerals

An ample and balanced diet is without a doubt the best way to ensure adequate nutrition. However, much scientific evidence suggests that complementing the diet with a daily multivitamin and mineral supplement is a sensible precaution to help avoid nutrient deficiencies that are common in older adults.

The Food and Nutrition Board established dietary standards for evaluating the nutritional requirements of groups of people. One group of people may be children, another group of people may be adults, and still another group may be the elderly. All of these groups have different nutritional needs. The dietary nutritional standards for a group are called Recommended Dietary Allowances (RDA). The RDA for a nutrient is based on the amount needed to *prevent* a deficiency. New Dietary Reference Intakes (DRI), determined by the Food and Nutrition Board of the Institute of Medicine, will soon replace the RDA. The DRIs represent a shift from preventing deficiency to decreasing the risk of chronic disease through nutrition. DRIs include levels that may reduce the risk of heart disease, osteoporosis, certain cancers, and other diet-related diseases.

DRIs include recommended intakes, adequate intakes, and tolerable upper-intake limits for vitamins and minerals. The recommended intake (RDA) is the average dietary intake level of a nutrient that prevents a deficiency in 97 to 98 percent of a group of people. The adequate intake (AI) is a value set as a goal for individual intake of nutrients that don't have an RDA. The tolerable upper-intake level (UL) is the highest level of a nutrient that most likely will not have an adverse effect on the health of 98 percent of a group of people.

Let's review the main vitamins and minerals and their functions in the body, then look at list of their RDAs or AIs and ULs for the adult group (age 19 to 70). Some vitamins, like the B-complex vitamins, are water-soluble, which means they are not stored in the body and must be taken daily because they are quickly eliminated in the urine. Fat-soluble vitamins, such as A, D, E, and K, are stored in the body and thus have a longer duration of action and more potential for toxicity.

Vitamins

- **Vitamin A (including provitamin A carotenoids):** It is composed of a group of chemicals derived from beta-carotene. It is required for normal vision, the immune system, and aids in the growth and maintenance of bones, cells, and skin.

- B-complex: It is composed of a group of B vitamins.
  B_1–**Thiamine:** It is useful in the production of red blood cells and is needed for the breakdown of carbohydrates and the health of the nervous system.
  B_2–**Riboflavin:** It is useful in energy production and is necessary for proper nerve maintenance and the maintenance of skin, hair, and nails.
  B_3–**Niacin:** It helps improve metabolism, improves the condition of the skin, and supports both the digestive and nervous systems.
  B_5–**Pantothenic acid:** It is involved in the generation of energy, production of blood cells, and the synthesis of bile, fats, and steroid hormones.
  B_6–**Pyridoxine:** It is involved in immune function, the nervous system and neurotransmitters, red blood cell production, and energy production.
  B_9–**Folic acid (folate):** It is essential for red blood cell formation and for the formation of DNA in general (the requirement for folic acid is greatest in rapidly dividing cells, such as blood cells).
  B_{12}–**Cyanocobalamin:** It is involved in blood cell formation and also essential for formation of nerve and spinal cord fibers.
  Biotin: Biotin is a member of the B-complex group of vitamins. Biotin is essential for the metabolism of protein and carbohydrates (like the other B vitamins) and for the production of hormones and cholesterol.

- **Choline:** It assists in maintenance of the nervous system and its neurotransmitters, gallbladder regulation, liver functions, and lecithin production.

- **Vitamin C**: Its antioxidant properties protect cell tissues from breakdown caused by free radical formation. It promotes the absorption of iron and the formation of bone, strengthens blood vessels, and supports the immune system. The water-soluble form is known as ascorbic acid. There is a fat-soluble form known as ascorbyl palmitate, which is better absorbed than ascorbic acid. It offers all the benefits of ascorbic acid, plus it won't flush out of the body as quickly as ascorbic acid, and it is able to be stored in cell membranes until the body needs it.

- **Vitamin D**: Vitamin D (cholecalciferol) is converted to an active form, called Vitamin D_3, in the upper layers of the skin. Technically, it is a hormone. This active form is essential for the formation of bone. It must be present in order for calcium to be absorbed from the intestine and ultimately be stored in your bone, and it also works with the parathyroid hormone to increase the storage of calcium in the bone. Individuals who are infrequently exposed to sunlight will have low levels of activated vitamin D and fragile bones.

  - **Sunlight for Bone Health**: Our bodies are specifically programmed to manufacture the exact amount of Vitamin D we need from the ultraviolet B rays (UVB) of sunlight. Vitamin D is converted to its active form in the upper layers of the skin when sunlight hits the skin. If there is enough sunlight to cause a reddening of your skin when you are outside for any length of time, then there are enough UVB rays to help your body make vitamin D. Generally, vitamin D reaches maximum levels in light skin twenty minutes after exposure (darkly pigmented skin requires a longer exposure, at least twice as long or longer, because this type of skin somewhat inhibits ultraviolet light from the sun). Early-morning or late-afternoon sunlight exposure is the safest. Avoid midday sun (from 10:00 A.M. to 3:00 P.M.) and sunburn.

    If you expose your face and hands to sunlight without sunscreen (that's right, *without* sunscreen because sunscreen blocks the skin reaction) for about twenty minutes three to four times per week for four to five months per year, you will probably get enough UVB rays to maintain your bone strength. Your body will store up vitamin D for use during low-sunlight times. The more skin you expose, the quicker you make vitamin D. So, some experts recommend full-body exposure for fifteen minutes. You are *not* sunbathing. If you plan on being in the sun longer than twenty minutes, apply sunscreen.

Beware of sunlight sensitivity and increased burning if you are taking antibiotics in the cycline and sulfa family, sulfonylurea diabetic medications, diuretics of the thiazide family, and Retin-A and Renova skin treatment products.

During the winter months or at higher latitudes, the sun is not high enough in the sky to stimulate vitamin D production. In the absence of sunlight, you must get the vitamin in your diet or with supplementation.

- **Vitamin E:** It is composed of a group of tocopherols, alpha-tocopherol being the main compound. It decreases free radical damage to cell tissues, speeds wound healing, reduces scar formation, and promotes healthy skin. Natural vitamin E contains alpha-tocopherol exclusively in an active form (either as d-alpha tocopherol or stabilized as d-alpha tocopheryl acid succinate, d-alpha-tocopheryl succinate, or d-alpha-tocopheryl acetate). Natural vitamin E may also contain other types of tocopherols, such as beta-tocopherol, delta-tocopherol, and gamma-tocopherol. Some manufacturers use the term "mixed" tocopherols when referring to these different types. Synthetic vitamin E (sometimes referred to as dl-alpha-tocopherol) contains both active and inactive forms of alpha-tocopherol. The Recommended Dietary Allowance (RDA) for vitamin E is based only on active alpha-tocopherol. Consequently the amount of vitamin E needed by individuals to meet the RDA is different for natural versus synthetic vitamin E.

- **Vitamin K:** It is essential for blood clotting and stored in the body. Normally, there is an ample store in the liver, and bacteria in the intestine also make vitamin K. It is readily available in green, leafy vegetables. This vitamin sometimes is in multivitamin and mineral supplements.

Minerals

Mineral supplements are used differently in the body than are vitamins. Most mineral supplements are essential metals and *trace* amounts are required for normal body function.

- **Boron** has no clear biological function in our bodies.

- **Calcium** is essential for proper muscle and nerve function, as well as for building bone.

- **Chromium** aids in the metabolism of sugars and maintenance of normal blood sugar levels.

- **Copper** is essential for proper blood formation.

- **Fluoride** inhibits the initiation and progression of dental caries and stimulates new bone formation.

- **Iodine** is essential for proper thyroid function.

- **Iron** is essential for red blood cell formation.

- **Magnesium** is essential for muscle function.

- **Manganese** is involved in bone formation and the enzymes involved in amino acid, cholesterol, and carbohydrate metabolism.

- **Molybdenum** promotes normal cell function. It enables the body to use nitrogen and is important for enzymes needed in metabolism. It also helps regulate iron stores in the body.

- **Nickel** has no clear biological function in our bodies.

- **Phosphorus** is essential for every cell in the body for normal function and is a major structural component of bone.

- **Potassium** is essential for proper heart and nerve function and for cellular stability.

- **Selenium** is essential for healthy immune system functioning and the thyroid gland. It is an important part of antioxidant enzymes that protect cells against the effects of free radicals that are produced during normal oxygen metabolism.

- **Silicon** has no clear biological function in our bodies.

- **Sodium** is essential for nerve and muscle function and for cellular stability. Sodium is plentiful in a variety of foods and is not supplemented.

- **Sulfur** is essential for energy production and cell function.

- **Vanadium** has no clear biological function in our bodies.

- **Zinc** is essential for proper immune function.

Recommended Amounts and Food Sources

The following vitamin and mineral chart contains the current RDA, and the newer RDA or AI requirements for adults (ages 19 to 70), upper tolerable limits, and food sources. Acronyms include IU/day, or International Units per day, g/day, or grams per day, mg/day, or milligrams per day, and mcg/day, or micrograms per day.

Vitamin	Current RDA	Adult Men's New RDA or AI	Adult Women's New RDA or AI	Tolerable Upper Limit (UL)	Select Food Sources
Vitamin A, includes provitamin A carotenoids	5000 IU/day	900 mcg/day or 3,000 IU/day	700 mcg/day or 2,333 IU/day	3,000 mcg/day or 10,000 IU/day	Liver, dairy products, fish, darkly colored fruits, and leafy vegetables
B₁–Thiamine	1.5 mg/day	1.2 mg/day	1.1 mg/day	Not determined, source should be from food only to prevent high levels of intake	Enriched, fortified, or whole-grain products; bread and bread products, mixed foods whose main ingredient is grain and ready-to-eat cereals
B₂–Riboflavin	1.7 mg/day	1.3 mg/day	1.1 mg/day	Not determined	Organ meats, milk, bread products, and fortified cereals
B₃–Niacin	20 mg/day	16 mg/day	14 mg/day	35 mg/day From synthetic forms of niacin obtained from supplements, fortified foods, or a combination of the two	Meat, fish, poultry, enriched and whole-grain breads and bread products, fortified ready-to-eat cereals
B₅–Pantothenic acid	10 mg/day	5 mg/day	5 mg/day	Not determined	Chicken, beef, potatoes, oats, cereals, tomato products, liver, kidney, yeast, egg yolk, broccoli, whole grains
B₆–Pyridoxine	2 mg/day	1.3 mg/day (age 19–50) 1.7 mg/day (age 50–70)	1.3 mg/day (age 19–50) 1.5 mg/day (age 50–70)	100 mg/day	Fortified cereals, organ meats, fortified soy-based meat substitutes

Vitamin	Current RDA	Adult Men's New RDA or AI	Adult Women's New RDA or AI	Tolerable Upper Limit (UL)	Select Food Sources
B_9–Folic acid (folate)	400 mcg/day	400 mcg/day	400 mcg/day	1,000 mg/day From synthetic supplement forms and/or fortified cereals	Enriched cereals, grains, dark leafy vegetables, enriched and whole-grain breads and bread products, fortified ready-to-eat cereals
B_{12}– Cyanocobalamin	6 mcg/day	2.4 mcg/day	2.4 mcg/day	Not determined	Fortified cereals, meat, fish, poultry
Vitamin C	60 mg/day	90 mg/day Smokers require an additional 35 mg/day. Nonsmokers regularly exposed to tobacco smoke should make sure they are meeting the RDA.	75 mg/day Smokers require an additional 35 mg/day. Nonsmokers regularly exposed to tobacco smoke should make sure they are meeting the RDA.	2,000 mg/day	Citrus fruits, tomatoes, tomato juice, potatoes, Brussels sprouts, cauliflower, broccoli, strawberries, cabbage, and spinach
Vitamin D (Calciferol)	10 mcg/day or 400 IU/day	5 mcg/day or 200 IU/day (age 19–50) 10 mcg/day or 400 IU/day (age 50–70)	5 mcg/day or 200 IU/day (age 19–50) 10 mcg/day or 400 IU/day (age 50–70)	50 mcg/day or 2,000 IU/day	Fish liver oils, flesh of fatty fish, liver, eggs, fortified milk products, and fortified cereals
Vitamin E	20 mg/day or 30 IU/day	15 mg/day or 22 IU/day for natural Vitamin E or 33 IU/day for synthetic Vitamin E	15 mg/day or 22 IU/day for natural Vitamin E or 33 IU/day for synthetic Vitamin E	1,000 mg/day or 1,500 IU/day from natural vitamin E or 2,200 IU/day from synthetic vitamin E From any alpha-tocopherol supplement form, fortified foods, or a combination of the two	Vegetable oils, unprocessed cereal grains, nuts, fruits, vegetables, and meats
Vitamin K	80 mcg/day	120 mcg/day	90 mcg/day	Not determined	Green vegetables, such as collards, spinach, salad greens, broccoli, Brussels sprouts, cabbage, plant oils
Biotin	300 mcg/day	30 mcg/day	30 mcg/day	Not determined	Liver and smaller amounts in fruits and vegetables
Choline There is not a sufficient body of evidence to assess whether a dietary supply of choline is needed at all.	Not established	550 mg/day	425 mg/day	3,500 mg/day	Milk, liver, eggs, peanuts

Vitamin	Current RDA	Adult Men's New RDA or AI	Adult Women's New RDA or AI	Tolerable Upper Limit (UL)	Select Food Sources
Minerals					
Calcium	1,000 mg/day	1,000 mg/day (age 19–50) 1,200 mg/day (age 50–70)	1,000 mg/day (age 19–50) 1,200 mg/day (age 50–70)	2,500 mg/day	Milk, cheese, yogurt, corn tortillas, calcium-set tofu, Chinese cabbage, kale, broccoli
Chromium	120 mcg/day	35 mcg/day (age 19–50) 30 mcg/day (age 50–70)	25 mcg/day (age 19–50) 20 mcg/day (age 50–70)	Not determined	Some cereals, meats, poultry, fish, beer
Copper	2 mg/day	900 mcg/day	900 mcg/day	10,000 mcg/day	Organ meats, seafood, nuts, seeds, wheat bran, cereals, whole-grain products, cocoa products
Iodine	150 mcg/day	150 mcg/day	150 mcg/day	1,100 mcg/day Individuals with thyroid conditions may not be protected by the UL for iodine intake for the general population.	Marine origin, processed foods, iodized salt
Iron Non-heme iron absorption is lower for those eating a vegetarian diet and it has been suggested that the iron requirement be twice as much. Recommended intake assumes 75% of iron is from heme iron sources.	18 mg/day	8 mg/day	18 mg/day (age 19–50) 8 mg/day (age 50–70)	45 mg/day	Fruits, vegetables, fortified bread and grain products, such as cereal (non-heme iron sources) and meat and poultry (heme iron sources)
Magnesium	400 mg/day	400 mg/day (age 19–30) 420 mg/day (age 30–70)	310 mg/day (age 19–30) 320 mg/day (age 30–70)	350 mg/day Limit is from supplement form only, does not include intake from food and water.	Green leafy vegetables, unpolished grains, nuts, meat, milk
Manganese	2 mg/day	2.3 mg/day	1.8 mg/day	11 mg/day	Nuts, legumes, tea, and whole grains Manganese in drinking water and supplements may be more absorbable than that from food.
Molybdenum	75 mcg/day	45 mcg/day	45 mcg/day	2,000 mcg/day	Legumes, grain products, and nuts
Phosphorus	1,000 mg/day	700 mg/day	700 mg/day	4,000 mg/day	Milk, yogurt, ice cream, cheese, peas, meat, eggs, some cereals and breads

Vitamin	Current RDA	Adult Men's New RDA or AI	Adult Women's New RDA or AI	Tolerable Upper Limit (UL)	Select Food Sources
Selenium	70 mcg/day	55 mcg/day	55 mcg/day	400 mcg/day	Organ meats, seafood, plant grown in selenium-rich soil
Zinc Zinc absorption is lower for those eating a vegetarian diet and it has been suggested that the zinc requirement be twice as much.	15 mg/day	11 mg/day	8 mg/day	40 mg/day	Fortified cereals, red meats, and certain seafood

Dietary Supplements

A dietary supplement is any product that is intended to supplement the diet and that contains at least one of these ingredients: vitamins, minerals, herbs or other botanicals, amino acids, and substances such as enzymes, organ tissues, glandulars, metabolites, or a combination of these ingredients. If you choose to take a dietary supplement, choose a good, general multivitamin, multi-mineral supplement. It should offer the full nutrient spectrum, including chromium, which helps insulin work more effectively, the full range of B-complex vitamins, and antioxidants like vitamins E and C and beta-carotene. Look at the source of the vitamin A and make sure that part or all of it comes from beta-carotene. A good rule of thumb is to look for daily value percentage ranges from 50 to 150 percent.

Read the supplement label carefully. It will show how much of a specific vitamin is in each multivitamin. If a multivitamin has some but not enough of the other vitamins, you can take additional doses of those particular single supplements. Typically, a multivitamin cannot hold enough calcium. Natural and synthetic vitamins are basically the same, except the natural form of vitamin E is considered easier for the body to assimilate. Also consider the name of the manufacturer or distributor. Nationally known food and drug manufacturers already have manufacturing standards in place, so their quality control may be better than that of lesser-known companies. Choose the most cost-effective formulation.

To help consumers make informed choices of supplements, the Food and Drug Administration (FDA) developed regulations for manufacturers. Manufacturers are responsible for ensuring that their supplements' facts label and ingredient list are accurate, that the dietary ingredients are safe, and that the content matches the amount declared on the label. Here is the information that must be on a dietary supplement label:

- A descriptive name of the product stating that it is a supplement.

- The name and address of the manufacturer, packager, or distributor.

- A list of each ingredient contained in the product, listed in the order of pre-dominance by common name or proprietary blend. Ingredients not listed on the facts panel must appear in the other ingredient statement beneath the panel. Other ingredients could include water, sweeteners, gelatin, starch, colors, stabilizers, preservatives, and flavorings.

- The net contents of the product.

  A supplement facts panel will show the following:

- The manufacturer's suggested serving size. There are no rules that limit a serving size or the amount of a nutrient in any form of dietary supplements.

- Information on nutrients when they are present in significant levels, such as vitamins A and C, calcium, iron, and sodium, and the percentage Daily Value (% DV) where a reference has been established—this is similar to the nutrients listed in the Nutrition Facts panel on food labels. The Daily Value is essentially the same as the DRI (RDA or AI). For example, if a nutrient's RDA is 60 mg (%DV is 100%), and this product has 200 mg, then this product's percentage Daily Value will be 333 percent (200mg/60mg) × 100).

- All other dietary ingredients present in the product, including botanicals and amino acids—those for which no Daily Value has been established.

Single Nutrient Supplementation

In addition to this basic multivitamin and mineral supplement, you may want to take single supplements to boost your health for specific conditions. To be sure that you will not be taking excessive amounts over what is already in the basic supplement, subtract the amount in the basic supplement from the larger amount listed for that single supplement. The difference is the amount of the single supplement you need to add. For example, if your basic supplement provides 200 mg of calcium, you would only take 800 mg of single supplement calcium to receive 1,000 mg of calcium daily.

For added antioxidant supplementation, which is especially important if you live in a polluted city, are taxed by daily stresses, are a vigorous daily exerciser, or are engaged in athletic competition, include the following in your diet:

- Up to 1,000 mg of vitamin C per day (Take these supplements in divided doses; vitamin C will saturate body tissues at doses between 120 and 200 mg. The excess is excreted in the urine. Higher doses tend to cause gastrointestinal distress.)

- 400 to 800 IU of Vitamin E per day

- 25,000 IU of mixed-carotenes (beta-carotene with related compounds, alpha-carotene, lutein, zeaxanthin) (Intakes of beta-carotene above 20 mg/day may turn the skin yellow, most notably the palms of the hands, the soles of the feet, and possibly the whites of the eye.)

- 200 to 300 mcg of selenium daily

- 100 mg of alpha lipoic acid twice daily

  For bone health, women should take:

- Between 1,000 and 1,500 mg of calcium citrate or carbonate plus 400 IU of vitamin D

- 500 mg magnesium (gluconate, chelate, or citrate) (Calcium and magnesium balance each other and vitamin D helps with calcium absorption.)

Take these supplements in divided doses with meals, because the body can absorb about a maximum of 750 mg of calcium at a time.

Common Herbal Supplements

These common herbal supplements are sometimes found in the formulation of high-potency or a health-benefit specific multivitamin and mineral supplement. Some herbs are used as *specifics*, taken for brief periods or only when symptoms are present. Some herbs are used as *tonics*, taken long term, sometimes with short breaks in between. For more information on using herbs and their health benefits, read about them from a reliable source (refer to Appendix C) and then discuss them with your health practitioner. Become informed!

- **Ginko Biloba (*Ginko Biloba*)** is an antioxidant and improves circulation and memory. It may interact with monoamine oxidase (MAO) inhibitors and blood-thinners and may cause gastrointestinal upset and headaches.

- **Gotu Kola (*Centella asiatica*)** improves circulation, healing and memory, and reduces stress.

- **Ginseng (*Panax ginseng, P. quinquefolius*)** helps increase energy, and is used as a tonic for fatigue and athletic performance. It may worsen the side effects of stimulants, such as caffeine. Some people experience over-stimulation or stomach upset when taking this herb. Do not take this herb if you have high blood pressure, heart palpitations, insomnia, asthma, or a high fever.

- **Siberian Ginseng or Eleuthero (*Eleuthero senticosus*)** helps increase energy and is used as a tonic for fatigue and stress. Its use may increase the effectiveness and side effects of some antibiotics.

- **Saw Palmetto (*Sernoa repens*)** is effective in the treatment of prostate enlargement (benign prostatic hyperplasia [BPH]). Some people experience stomach upset when taking this herb.

- **Echinacea (*Echinacea augustifolia, E. pallida, E. Purpurea*)** is known for its ability to stimulate the body's defenses against minor vial and bacterial infections such as colds and the flu. Persons allergic to the pollen of other members of the aster family, such as ragweed, may also be allergic to echinacea. Its use may counteract immune-suppressive drugs.

- **Astragalus (*Astragalus membranaceus*)** is known for its immune-boosting, antiviral, antibacterial, and tonic properties and is used for colds, the flu, and minor infections.

- **Grapeseed Extract (*Vitis vinifera*)** is also known as pycnogenol. It has anti-oxidant compounds that inhibit swelling and inflammation.

- **Green Tea Extract (*Camellia Sinensis* plant extract)** has antioxidant properties (namely the phytochemical epigallocatechin gallate [EGCG]) and is used as a tonic.

- **Garlic (*Allium sativum*)** has antiviral and antibacterial properties, and studies have shown that it lowers cholesterol. Its use may increase the effects of blood-thinners.

- **Milk Thistle (*Silybum marianum*)** is a liver protector and healer and is used as a liver tonic.

- **Bilberry (*Vaccinium myrtillus*)** has antioxidant properties and improves circulation.

- **Black Cohosh (*Cimicifuga racemosa*)** has been shown to be effective for premenstrual and menopausal symptoms, such as hot flashes. It may cause stomach upset. Pregnancy and nursing women should avoid using this herb.

Supplement Safety

When taking dietary supplements, it is important to fully inform your health care provider about the vitamins, minerals, herbals, or any other supplements you are taking. Dietary supplements may not be risk-free under certain circumstances. If you plan to use a dietary supplement in place of drugs or in combination with any drug, discuss your plans with your health care provider first. Many supplements contain active ingredients that have strong biological effects and their safety is not always assured for all users. If you have certain health conditions and take these products, you may be placing yourself at risk.

Some supplements may interact with prescription and over-the-counter medicines. Taking a combination of supplements or using these products together with medications (whether prescription or over-the-counter [OTC] drugs) could under certain circumstances produce adverse effects, some of which could be life-threatening. Some supplements may produce undesirable effects such as fatigue, diarrhea, and hair loss when taken in large amounts. Too much of one mineral can interfere with the absorption of other minerals you may need.

Also some supplements can have unwanted effects during surgery. You may be asked to stop taking these products at least two to three weeks before the procedure to avoid potentially dangerous supplement and drug interactions—such as changes in heart rate and blood pressure, and increased bleeding—that could adversely affect the outcome of your surgery.

4

A Reasonable Eating Plan

The easiest path to good nutrition is to eat a variety of foods. Food nourishes us by supplying our bodies with protein, carbohydrates, fats, fiber, water, anti-oxidants, anti-inflammatories, vitamins, and minerals. Eating fewer processed and packaged foods, such as crackers, cookies and cakes, and increasing your intake of fiber-rich, nutrient-dense foods is a good way to start and maintain good nutrition. The secret for eating a well-balanced, healthy diet is to eat a wide assortment of foods, which ensures that you include all the nutrients you need. And it's not just about eating nutritious foods; it's also about the amount of those foods that you eat. In choosing a variety of foods, it is important to know how much of those foods to eat—in other words, what are the reasonable serving sizes. Being able to judge food portions will help you in planning meals at home and in dining out. It is important to wean yourself from a Super-Size mentality.

A reasonable eating plan to improve your health involves:

- **Planning Serving Sizes:** Learn how food product Nutrition Facts labels can help you select a food and the serving size. Find out what standard serving and portion sizes are and how to determine serving and portion sizes of foods and meals

- **Selecting Nourishing Foods:** Choose highly nourishing foods that provide the necessary proteins, fats, carbohydrates, fiber, and water for health when planning and creating meals.

- **Building Meals:** Create your own meals at home and meals to choose when eating out.

- **Supplementing Your Plan:** Take daily dietary supplements to ensure that you are getting all the vitamins, minerals, and other vital nutrients. Practicing good dental health will add to your overall healthy lifestyle.

Purchase a calorie, fat, and carbohydrate or carbohydrate-counter pocket diet guide to help you understand portion sizes. These little books are chockfull of nutritional information. Some guides have an added bonus, a fast food and restaurant section, which helps you make healthier, wiser food choices while dining out.

Planning Serving Sizes

The Nutrition Facts label on food products makes it easy for you to know what is in the food you eat. Sections on the label consist of Serving Size Information, Amount of Calories per Serving and Calories from Fat, a Nutrition Panel, and a Nutrition Reference footnote panel. The Nutrition Panel lists nutrients that are most important to the health of people today, such as Total Fat (grams), Saturated Fat (grams), Polyunsaturated Fat (grams), Monounsaturated Fat (grams), Cholesterol (milligrams), Sodium (milligrams), Potassium (milligrams), Total Carbohydrate (grams), Dietary Fiber (grams), Sugars (grams), and Protein (grams). The Percentage Daily Value shows you the percentage (or how much) of the recommended dietary amount of a nutrient is in one serving of the food based on the nutrition values in the Nutrition Reference footnote. The Percentage Daily Values (% Daily Value) of each amount are based on a 2,000-calorie diet. The Percentage Daily Values of the vitamins and minerals are based on the Food and Nutrition Board's Recommended Dietary Allowances (RDA). For example, if a product has listed the % Daily Value for vitamin C as 2 percent and the RDA is 60 mg, then this product is providing 12 mg of vitamin C (0.002 multiplied by 60 mg equals 1.2 mg). Another example, if calcium is listed as 30 percent and the RDA is 1,000 mg, and then this product provides 300 mg. (Chapter 3 has a chart of the RDAs.)

The Nutrition Reference footnote has nutritional data for Total Fat and types of fat such as Saturated, Cholesterol, Sodium, Total Carbohydrate, and Dietary Fiber based on a diet that is approximately 60 percent carbohydrates, 30 percent fats, and 10 percent protein. It lists the data for a 2,000-calorie-a-day diet and a 2,500-calorie-a-day diet. Data on this footnote do not change from food product to food product; it shows dietary advice.

The Nutrition Facts label's serving unit is *specific for each product category* and designed to help consumers compare nutritional information on a number of foods within a category. The label serving size is not meant to tell you *how much to eat* but to help you identify nutrients in a food and to make product comparisons easier. The Nutrition Facts label's serving units cover a range of mixed products, from frozen food entrées to simple food items.

Here's how to use the information on these labels to make wise decisions on portion size. Say, for example, that an 11.5-ounce can of vegetable juice states that the serving size is 1 can, the number of calories for this serving is 70, and the total carbohydrate amount is 15 grams. If you were reducing your carbohydrate intake, you could drink half of the serving amount, taking in 35 calories with 7.5 grams of carbohydrates. Now, what about a 20-ounce bottle of a soft drink? The number of calories per serving shows about 140 calories. However, the serving size is 2.5 servings. If you drink the entire bottle, you've taken in 350 calories! This may not be the caloric amount you had in mind if you thought the whole bottle was one serving! Look at the Nutrition Facts label to learn the *size* of the serving and the *number* of servings.

Standard Serving Sizes

The U.S. Department of Agriculture's (USDA) *Dietary Guidelines for Americans* sets forth serving size standards based on typical portion sizes and the nutritional content of foods. It describes serving *units* for each food group, such as ½ cup cooked vegetables and 1 cup raw leafy vegetables, to make it easy for consumers to make healthful food choices. These servings units cover simple food items, such as fruits, vegetables, and plain grain products.

Generally, standard serving sizes are as follows:

Grain Products (bread, cereal, rice, and pasta)

- 1 slice of bread

- 1 ounce of ready-to-eat cereal

- ½ cup of cooked cereal, rice, or pasta

Vegetables and Fruits

- 1 cup of raw leafy vegetables

- ½ cup of other vegetables—cooked or chopped raw

- ¾ cup of vegetable juice

- 1 medium apple, banana, orange

- ½ cup of chopped, cooked, or canned fruit

- ¾ cup of fruit juice

Protein (meat, poultry, fish, dry beans, eggs, and nuts) and Dairy (milk, yogurt, and cheese)

- 2–3 ounces of cooked lean meat, poultry, or fish

- ½ cup of cooked dry beans or 1 egg counts as 1 ounce of lean meat; 2 tablespoons of peanut butter or 1/3 cup of nuts count as 1 ounce of meat

- 1 cup of milk or yogurt

- 1½ ounces of natural cheese

- 2 ounces of processed cheese

For many food items, the serving size in the Dietary Guidelines and on the Nutrition Facts label is the same, for example, ½ cup canned fruits or vegetables. However, some serving sizes differ because the Dietary Guidelines and the Nutrition Facts label serve different purposes. Many Dietary Guidelines serving sizes are smaller that those on the Nutrition Facts label. For example, on the Nutrition Facts label, one serving of cooked cereal, rice, or pasta is 1 cup, but the serving size standard is only ½ cup.

In both cases, serving size is a unit of measure and may not be the portion of food that you actually eat. A grilled cheese sandwich is a good example; it is a portion made up of two servings of bread and one serving of cheese. A fast-food cheeseburger with lettuce and tomato could be a portion that is made up of two servings of bread, one serving of vegetables, one serving of meat, and one serving of cheese. Even though, serving size and portion size are used interchangeably. Generally, a portion of food is the amount of specific food you eat for a meal or a snack. Portions can be larger or smaller than the servings listed in the Dietary Guidelines or on the Nutrition Facts label. Using portion size measuring methods will enable you to enjoy sensible dining.

Determining Food Serving Sizes

It is so easy to overestimate how much food makes up a serving size. The most important thing is to be able to eyeball portion sizes and know how much you are really eating. There are three methods that may work for you: the comparison method, the pre-measured method, and the hand method.

1. Comparison Method: Compare how much of what you are eating with a familiar object. Here are a few comparisons:

1 ounce cheese	A pair of dice
3 ounces of meat	A deck of cards
½ cup mashed potatoes	An ice cream scoop
1 medium potato	A computer mouse
½ cup serving of grapes	A light bulb
1 serving of fruit	A tennis ball
1 serving of pasta	A hockey puck
1 serving of bread	A cassette tape
1 tablespoon of peanut butter	A walnut
¼ cup serving	A golf ball
2 ½ ounce bagel	Length of a credit card
6 ounces of juice	Small yogurt container

2. Pre-Measured Method: Using a set of measuring spoons, a glass measuring cup for liquids, a set of measuring cups for dry foods, and a kitchen scale for weighing raw fruits and vegetables, meat, and cheese, you pre-measure all your food portions. You will be surprised to see the actual amount of a serving size of food on your dinner plate or in your cereal bowl. You may want to use smaller plates and bowls to reduce the psychological impact of feeling that you are not eating enough food!

Weigh meat, poultry, and fish after cooking. In restaurants, the menu lists the precooked weight of the meat, so use this conversion rule to convert raw weight into cooked weight:

- Meat with bone: 5 raw ounces equals 3 ounces cooked (a standard serving size is 3 ounces).

- Meat without bone: 4 raw ounces equals 3 ounces cooked.

Examples of pre-measured quantities:

Bagel

Small	2 ounces
Medium	3 ounces
Large	4 ounces

Bread Roll

Small	1.5 ounces
Medium	1.8 ounces
Large	2.7 ounces
Extra large	4.5 ounces

Grapes

Small bunch	4 ounces
Large bunch	8 ounces
Extra-large bunch	16 ounces

Bananas

Small	5 ounces

Medium	6 ounces
Large	8 ounces

3. Hand Method: Use your hand to gauge portion size. Here are some approximate measurements based on an average-size woman's hand:

Thumb volume	1 ounce or 1 tablespoon Good estimate for nut butter, spreads and dips, mayonnaise, oils, salad dressings, sour cream, cream cheese
Thumb tip	1 teaspoon
Finger length	Diameter of 1 serving of fruit
Fist volume (clenched fist)	1 cup or 2 servings of pasta, cereal, cooked vegetables, or 1 serving of raw vegetables
Palm area	3-ounce serving of meat, fish, poultry
Handful	1 serving of nuts
Two handfuls	1 serving of most snack foods

Selecting Nourishing Foods

The number of servings suggested depends on your calorie needs. For example, inactive women and some older adults may need around 1,600 calories per day, while active women and inactive men may need about 2,200 calories per day and active men may need around 2,800 calories. Choose the lesser amount of the suggested servings if you have lower caloric needs, and choose the mid-level or higher amount if you have higher caloric needs.

1. Beverages

Water
Green tea, hot or iced
Coffee, hot or iced
Vegetable juice
Occasional glass (4 to 6 ounces) of red wine with dinner (not daily)

If you drink coffee and want to drink more green tea instead, but you love the roasted flavor of coffee, try Kukicha twig tea. This is a Japanese green tea in which the tea leaves and twigs have been roasted slowly and repeatedly. This tea is greatly appreciated in Japan for its mellowness.

Note: You need to be drinking at least eight or more 8-ounce glasses of fluid a day.

Use Moderation When Drinking Alcohol

On those occasions when you drink alcohol, keep in mind that moderation is the key! Moderation is defined as no more than one drink per day for women and no more than two drinks per day for men. This limit is because of differences between the sexes in both weight and metabolism.

Count as one drink:

- 12 ounces of regular beer (150 calories)

- 5 ounces of wine (100 calories)

- 1.5 ounces of 80 proof distilled spirits (liquor) (100 calories)

2. Protein Foods

Choose 3 to 4 servings daily
One serving from

Beef, pork, fish, poultry, tofu   Remember 1 serving is the
Includes canned fish, tuna, salmon, sar-   size of a deck of cards!
dines, herring, vegetable protein burger

Or

Dried beans, peas, lentils or legumes (black, chickpeas, kidney, lima, butter, navy, pinto, soy)	½ cup

Or

Soy milk	1 cup

Or

Raw nuts and seeds	A little over 2 tablespoons

Or

Yogurt, cottage cheese, ricotta, cheese	½ cup yogurt, cottage or ricotta cheese 2 diced-size pieces of cheese (1 ounce)

Or

Eggs	1 egg

Select cured meats (bacon, salami, lunchmeats, and hot dogs) on occasion and minimize their portion size. They are high in nitrates and nitrites.
Select shellfish on occasion. Not all shellfish comes from clean waters.

3. Choosing Fat

Besides the small amount of fat that is used in cooking your foods, include flaxseed oil or olive oil daily for your omega-3 and omega-9 essential fatty acid (EFA) needs.

For Your Omega-3 EFA Needs

If you don't care for fish, you can take a tablespoon of flaxseed oil a day or a tablespoon of flaxseed meal sprinkled over your food (cereal, salad, cooked vegetables). Keep in mind that the oil has about 130 calories per tablespoon, so adjust your total daily caloric intake accordingly, and flaxseed meal is high in fiber and it may have a laxative effect in some people. You can find flaxseed oil, in the refrigerator section, and flaxseeds and flaxseed meal (preground flaxseed) in a natural foods store or the specialty (sometimes organic or health) foods section of your supermarket. You can make flaxseed meal fresh by grinding the whole seeds, a half-cup at a time, in a coffee grinder. Store the freshly ground meal in the refrigerator.

For Your Omega-9 EFA Needs

Up to 12 percent of your total calories should come from monounsaturated fats. Olive oil has a high ratio of monounsaturated fat in the form of oleic acid and contains omega-9, omega-6, and some omega-3. The daily requirement for these fatty acids is supplied by 2 to 3 tablespoons of olive oil per day. Also, 1 tablespoon of olive oil provides 8 percent of the daily requirement for vitamin E.

4. Choosing Carbohydrates

Make low-carbohydrate (slow-acting carbohydrates) foods the mainstay of your diet, but limit their portion size for weight control.

Vegetables:

Choose five to eight servings of vegetables daily. Remember a serving size is ½ cup cooked and 1 cup raw.

Choose these slow-acting carbohydrates that are slowly digested and absorbed to help maintain blood sugar levels. These vegetables are rich in antioxidants and minerals. Choose fresh greens, and the other vegetables fresh or frozen. Canned vegetables tend to be higher in salt, so if you are watching your sodium intake, avoid these.

Greens to select from are collard greens, kale, mustard greens, beet greens, spinach, Swiss chard, sorrel, purslane, savoy cabbage, green cabbage, red cabbage, Chinese cabbage, bok choy, romaine, red and green leaf lettuce, escarole, arugula, Belgian and curly endive, radicchio, and watercress. Also, select from broccoli, broccoli rabe, Brussels sprouts, cauliflower, asparagus, avocado, bell peppers (all color varieties), zucchini, summer squash, tomatoes, green beans, celery, cucumbers, eggplant, and lima beans.

Select the following items in condiment sizes (around 2 tablespoons), raw or fresh, lightly cooked, or use as seasonings: parsley and cilantro, garlic, onions, mushrooms (particularly shiitake, maitake, enokidake, oyster), ginger, turmeric, and olives.

Choose the quicker-acting carbohydrate vegetables only once or twice a week. Keep these to a minimum. These foods raise blood sugar levels more rapidly. Select corn, white and sweet potatoes, yams, green peas, beets, carrots, parsnips, rutabaga, and pumpkin.

Fruit:

Choose three to four servings of fruit daily. Remember a serving size is ½ cup sliced or one medium-size (remember the tennis ball?) whole fruit. Serving size is important when eating fruit! These fruits are rich in antioxidants and nutrients. Eat fruit when it is in season. For fruit such as berries; buy extra while they're in season and freeze for eating when the season is over: blueberries, strawberries, raspberries, blackberries, cherries, kiwi, plums, peaches, pears, apples, citrus fruits (grapefruit, lemons, oranges), and grapes.

Higher-carbohydrate fruits that you want to limit include watermelon, overripe bananas, cantaloupe, honeydew melon, pineapple, mango, guava, and papaya.

Grains:

Choose three to four servings daily. Remember that one serving of bread is one slice, one serving of cooked cereal, pasta, or grain is 1 cup. If you are reducing your carbohydrate intake, you may not want to eat grain products.

Because of their fiber content, whole-grain breads, sourdough bread, bran and oat (oatmeal, old-fashioned) cereals, barley, buckwheat, bulgur (kasha), pasta, and basmati rice can be considered slow-acting carbohydrates. Low-fiber cereals, crisp bread, and rye crisp crackers are high-carbohydrate foods; please eat a minimum!

Building Meals

From your healthful food selections, you build your daily meals. The following menus are just a sampling of nutritious meals that you can make and eat at home. There are a great many cookbooks and meal-planning books on the market. If you don't already own one, invest in one and be creative in your planning of nutritious, creative meals!

Breakfast

Brewed green or black tea or coffee, decaffeinated if you prefer
½ cup fruit or vegetable juice or 8 ounces of water

- Hot or cold whole-grain cereal, low-fat milk or soy milk, a medium piece of fruit or ½ cup of berries or sliced fruit

- 1 cup of plain yogurt mixed with 1 tablespoon of flaxseed meal or oil, ½ cup of berries, and a small bit of honey, maple syrup, or Splenda to sweeten

- 2 slices of whole grain toast with 1½ teaspoons of nut butter, such as peanut, soy or almond, and a medium piece of fruit

- Ricotta cheese mixed with a small amount of chopped walnuts, sliced fruit, and a small bit of your favorite sweetener

- Scrambled eggs with picante salsa, two strips of nitrate-free bacon or links of nitrate-free sausage

Lunch

8 ounces of water or brewed green or black tea

- Tuna fish salad and whole-grain bread sandwich, large tossed green salad with olive oil and lemon juice or vinegar

- Grilled chicken Caesar salad with dressing on the side, a medium piece of fresh fruit

- Vegetable, black bean, or lentil soup, sliced turkey and whole-grain bread sandwich with leafy lettuce, tomato, cheese, and bit of mayonnaise

- Cottage cheese with a large peach split in half served on green lettuce leaves, a crisp rye cracker

- Pasta with marinara sauce, tossed green salad with dressing on the side, gelato

Dinner

8 ounces of water or brewed green or black tea

- Grilled salmon or cold-water fish; grilled vegetables such as red, yellow, and green peppers, red onions, zucchini or summer squash; and basmati rice

- Spaghetti with marinara sauce in olive oil, steamed broccoli, tossed green salad

- Pasta with sautéed Swiss chard, steamed or sautéed vegetables, mixed fruit compote

- Broiled or grilled boneless, skinless chicken breast, steamed broccoli sprinkled with 1 tablespoon grated Parmesan cheese, a whole-grain roll

- Sirloin beef tips over noodles, steamed green beans, sliced strawberries

- Red beans and rice with salsa, tossed green salad with Greek olives

- Lentil soup, mixed vegetables, fresh fruit

Snacks (between breakfast and lunch, lunch and dinner, and after dinner):

8 ounces of water with each snack meal

- Apple slices with nut butter or a slice of hard cheese

- A hard-boiled egg

- Celery, carrot sticks, or pita chips with hummus

- Small handful of walnuts or pumpkin seeds

- Air-popped popcorn or low-fat microwave popcorn

Eating Out

You can make healthful food choices when dining out. You just need to be food aware. Here is a point to keep in mind. Some nutritionists suggest following an 80/20 rule, that is, eating a variety of nutritious foods 80 percent of the time and indulging in those wickedly delicious, but unhealthful foods, 20 percent of the time. If your diet is consistently nutritious, then eating the occasional hot dog or ice cream bar isn't going to affect you adversely.

Many fast-food chains and restaurants provide nutritional information for their customers at the establishment or on their Web sites. This information can help you make a healthful food choice when your only eating choice is at a restaurant. Some pocket calorie, fat, and carbohydrate counter guides have a section on the most popular fast-food chains and restaurants. Keeping one with you will increase your ability to choose more healthful foods when dining out. The book *Restaurant Confidential* also contains the amount of calories, sodium, fat, and much more for many popular restaurants.

Many, if not most, restaurants serve oversize portions, which equate to extra food and an increased amount of calories, fat, cholesterol, and sodium. A 10-inch plate of spaghetti is not a single serving size of ½ cup. To keep your portion sizes at a reasonable level:

- Order menu items a la carte. This gives you a variety of foods in smaller quantities.

- Ask if you can have a lunch portion, even if you're eating dinner. Or simply request a smaller portion.

- Split a meal with a companion, particularly when you know the restaurant serves larger portions.

- Request a to-go container when the meal arrives. Immediately place half of the food into the container for another day's meal.

- Eat only until your hunger is satisfied. If you're tempted to clean your plate, ask your server to remove the dishes.

At Restaurants

Read through the menu and select the items that are lower in saturated fat and calories. Read the description of the menu item. If none is available, ask your server what's in the meal and how it's prepared. Choose dishes based on fruits, vegetables, and whole grains rather than those based on meat. Plant-based foods are naturally low in fat and calories and are good sources of vitamins, minerals, and fiber. Fish and seafood also are good meal options.

You can find healthful options within each course of the meal. Here's how to do it:

Appetizers: Choose appetizers with vegetables, fruits, or fish. Tomato juice, fresh fruit compote, and shrimp cocktail served with lemon are healthful options. Avoid fried or breaded appetizers.

Soup: Choose broth-based or tomato-based soups, such as minestrone, vegetable, or gazpacho. Creamed soups, chowders, puréed soups and sometimes fruit soups can contain heavy cream or egg yolks. Ask your server for the soup's ingredients to find out for sure.

Salad: Order lettuce or spinach salad with dressing on the side, preferably oil and vinegar or vinaigrette. Caesar, Greek, and taco salads tend to be higher in fat and calories. Similarly, chef's salads can be high in fat, cholesterol, and calories because of the added dressing, cheese, eggs, and meat.

Bread: Choose whole-grain breads, rolls, breadsticks, crackers, or bagels. Muffins, garlic toast, and croissants have more calories and fat. If you have a basket of bread at your table, take one piece and ask your server to remove the basket. Use only small amounts of added fat—such as margarine, butter, or olive oil—or none at all.

Side dish: Choose steamed or sautéed vegetables rather than a baked potato, boiled new potatoes, or rice. Skip the French fries, potato chips, onion rings, or mayonnaise-based salads. Ask that the vegetables be served without butter or cream sauces.

Entrée: Look for descriptions that indicate lower-fat preparations, such as London broil, grilled chicken breast, lemon-baked fish, or broiled shish kebabs. Avoid items with high-fat descriptors, such as prime rib of beef, veal parmigiana, stuffed shrimp, fried chicken, fettuccine Alfredo, filet mignon with béarnaise sauce, shrimp tempura, or fried rice. Choose pasta primavera or linguine with red tomato or clam sauce. Skip pasta with meat or cheese stuffing or sauces that contain bacon, butter, cream, or eggs.

Dessert: Finish the main meal before ordering dessert. By the time you're done, you may not even want dessert. If you do order dessert, split it with your companions or take half of it home. Tasty and healthful dessert options include fresh fruit, gelatin, angel food cake, sorbet, or sherbet.

Beverages: Many soft drinks contain a large number of calories. Instead, order water, unsweetened iced tea, sparkling water, or mineral water with a twist of lemon. For a hot drink, try black, decaffeinated coffee or black or green tea, minus the sugar and other extras. Remember, too, that alcohol also contains many calories, and it may further stimulate your appetite and decrease your inhibitions about overeating. Enjoy these drinks in moderation.

Chinese, Italian, and Mexican Meal Choices

Watch out for high sodium and saturated fat in these meals. Make your selections from some of the popular dishes that have lower sodium and saturated fat.

Chinese choices:

- Steamed rice instead of fried-rice with your meals (½ cup rice is a serving size)
- Szechuan shrimp, without peanuts
- Stir-fried vegetables, shrimp with garlic sauce
- Vegetable lo mein
- Chicken chow mein
- Beef and broccoli

Italian choices (if you are choosing pasta, rather than broiled or grilled meat):

- A salad with half the dressing, if the dressing is served over the salad
- Minestrone and fagioli soups
- Spaghetti with marinara (tomato sauce) or meat sauce
- Linguini with red clam or white clam sauce

Mexican choices:

- Garden salad, with dressing on the side
- Jicama salad with vinaigrette
- Chicken, shrimp, or vegetable fajitas, without the beans, sour cream, and guacamole
- Grilled fish or chicken with tomatillo sauce

At Buffets

With buffets, large amounts of food and the freedom to go back for a second or third helping may lead to excess. To limit the amount of food you eat, survey the entire buffet line, and then decide what you want and take only that. Make salad minus the high-fat dressings and toppings, such as cheese and croutons, your first course. Then, go back for an entrée. Fill up on vegetables that don't have added butter or sauces.

At Fast-Food Restaurants

The nutritional value of fast foods, from cheeseburger to leanburgers to pizzas to tacos, can vary greatly. The majority of fast foods are high in calories, saturated fat, cholesterol, sodium, and sugar. Fried foods such as French fries and crispy chicken breasts are high in fat. However, fast-food restaurants are expanding their food choices to include healthy foods such as salads, salad bars, low-fat meat, whole-wheat breads, low-carbohydrate sandwiches, low-fat sandwiches, low-fat milk products, low-calorie foods, and vegetable oils. Avoid condiments such as special sauces, mayonnaise, cheese sauce, salad dressing, tartar sauce, and ketchup. They are high in fat and sugar. Some healthy food choices include:

- Grilled chicken
- Whole-wheat rolls
- Fruit or fruit and yogurt
- Salad with dressing on the side or fat-free salad dressing
- Single hamburger (regular or children's size)
- Low-fat deli sandwiches on wheat bread or on pita bread
- Wraps on whole-wheat tortillas without the dressing
- Water or low-fat milk

At a Pizza Chain

Some dietitians claim that pizza is a nutritious meal by itself, because it contains a grain, vegetable, dairy, and meat product. But it also comes with a high saturated fat count. The typical serving size of pizza varies from two slices to three slices, or approximately 9 ounces, depending on the restaurant and type of pizza. Make your selections from some of the popular pizza toppings that have lower sodium and saturated fat:

- Select vegetable toppings.

- If you must have meat, select chicken or ham. If not chicken or ham, make pepperoni your next choice; it is leaner than pork, sausage, and beef.

- Order your pizza with half the cheese or no cheese. Skip the extra cheese.

- Order a salad to go along with your pizza. Ask for the dressing on the side.

At the Airport

Airports can be stressful places. Eat because you're hungry, not because you're stressed, bored, or trying to kill time. If you're anxious or have time to spare, take a walk. Airports usually have plenty of room for a brisk walk. Here are some pointers:

- **Check out your dining options.** There are a lot more options, with more healthful choices. Skip the hot dog and pizza counters and look for eateries that serve fruit, soup, sushi, and sandwiches or wraps.

- **Order ahead.** If your flight includes a meal, request a special diet when you make your reservation. You might be able to choose a low-salt or low-fat option, or a diet or vegetarian plate. And when the beverage cart rolls your way, ask for water or juice instead of alcohol or soda.

- **Go Prepared.** Take along your own food if you're leaving or arriving very early or late when eateries are likely to be closed. You don't have to pack a picnic. A whole-wheat bagel or crackers, a piece of fruit, granola bar, juice box, or cut-up cheese and vegetables can save you from feeling starved.

At the Office

If you only have fifteen minutes for lunch between meetings, skip the vending machine. Keep your desk drawer stocked with nutritious foods that contribute to a healthy diet. When stocking your drawer, consider office foods that don't require refrigeration and can keep well for a month or so:

- Soup you can microwave

- Nuts and seeds

- Whole grain, low-fat crackers (Melba toast, Wasa, low-fat Triscuits)

- Whole-wheat pretzels

- Cheese and cracker snack packs

- Microwavable low-fat popcorn

- Granola bars

- Applesauce in cups

- Juice boxes (100% juice, vitamin C-rich, or vegetable juice)

Keep some take-out menus from nearby restaurants in your office for when you have to work late or have a little more time for lunch.

In the Car

Keep some of the same snacks you have in your office in your car. When you're dashing from one activity to another or stuck in traffic, they come in handy.

Following a Low-Carbohydrate Eating Plan

Select chicken or tuna salad, turkey, roast beef, and cheese in sandwich shops. Avoid the salami, bologna, and other meat products with nitrates. In fried chicken restaurants, avoid anything barbecued or breaded. Scrape the breading off, if you must. Select a grilled chicken sandwich instead. At salad bars, avoid any prepared dressings; use vinegar and oil. Avoid coleslaws and other prepared vegetable salads, including pasta salads. If you are at a pizza restaurant, order a salad or eat the topping off your pizza, leaving the crust. Avoid temptation by staying out of Mexican-style fast-food restaurants, doughnut shops, and yogurt or ice cream shops.

Supplementing Your Plan

Take a Multivitamin and Mineral Supplement

Subtle vitamin deficiencies can result from excessive consumption of nutrient-depleted foods such as refined sugar and white flour, from inadequate intake of vitamin-rich fruits and vegetables, and from nutrient losses due to processing, prolonged heating, or storage of foods. Sometimes you won't be eating whole, unprocessed foods that contain a wide array of beneficial substances besides vitamins, such as carotenoids, flavonoids, and natural antioxidants. You'll be eating at restaurants and fast-food chains. Remember, vitamin supplementation is not an adequate substitute for a good diet. The best approach to disease prevention is to eat properly *and* to take a multivitamin.

Practice Good Dental Health

What does your dental health have to do with healthier eating? The teeth and gums are the gateway to our digestive systems. Poor nutrition can result from inflamed gums and decayed teeth. Many of the foods that help your body build strong muscles and bones also help build strong, healthy teeth and gums. Dairy products provide calcium and vitamin D for strengthening teeth and bones. Breads and cereals supply B vitamins for growth and iron for healthy blood, which in turn contributes to healthy gum tissue. Lean meat, fish, poultry, and beans provide iron and protein for overall good health, and magnesium and zinc for strong teeth and bones. Fruits and vegetables containing antioxidants and anti-inflammatory compounds are essential to maintaining healthy gums. Recent research indicates that the phytochemicals, catechins, in green tea have compounds that have antibacterial properties. They are effective against *Streptococcus mutans*, the bacteria responsible for both decay and gum disease. Also, hard cheeses, especially cheddar, neutralize decay-causing acids that are produced by oral bacteria in the presence of other foods. Studies indicate that black tea may protect against periodontal disease. Black tea also contains fluoride, which protects against tooth decay.

Periodontal disease and tobacco use can both lead to tooth loss.

- **Periodontal disease** is a bacterial infection. Gingivitis is the mildest form of periodontal disease. There is evidence that infections in the mouth may lead to chronic diseases such as heart disease and stroke, besides leading to tooth loss. Dental professionals have long suspected this. Periodontal bacteria can enter the bloodstream and travel to major organs and begin new infections. Research is suggesting that this may contribute to the development of heart disease and increase the risk of stroke, increase a woman's risk of having a preterm, low-birth-weight baby, and pose a serious threat to people whose health is compromised by diabetes, respiratory diseases, or osteoporosis.

- **Use of any tobacco product,** whether smoked or chewed, can increase your risk of developing oral cancer and gum disease. Tobacco damages your oral structures by loosening the attachments between bone, tissue, and teeth, causing receding gums.

Even if you've managed to avoid periodontal disease until now, it is especially important to practice a meticulous oral care routine as you age. Receding gum tissue affects a large percentage of older people. This condition exposes the roots of teeth and makes them more vulnerable to decay and periodontal infection. If your poor dental health results in your getting dentures to replace missing teeth, you've introduced a new set of problems in your nutrition health. Denture wearers with full dentures, those that replace your entire set of teeth, uppers and lowers, may suffer more. Gum ridges in the mouth support dentures. Some denture wearers are never quite able to get a denture that has good suction to the gum tissues because of the shape of their gum tissues under the denture. As you get older, the bones under the gum ridges flatten, making it difficult for a dentist to make dentures that will have good suction to these gum ridges. These dentures will be looser when the person talks (that *click, click* you sometimes hear) or chews with the denture in place. Loose-fitting dentures also cause gum irritation. So, your mouth hurts, certain types of foods are now difficult to chew, the food seems to have lost its taste, and poor nutrition results.

Keep Your Teeth for a Lifetime

To keep your teeth for a lifetime, follow these simple guidelines:

- Be sensible, flexible, and realistic when making food choices. These are good rules for oral health as well as for nutrition.

- Drink green tea for its antioxidant and anti-inflammatory protection.

- Visit your dentist regularly for checkups, cleaning, and tooth restoration.

- Between visits, take care of your teeth, gums, and other soft tissues in the mouth as recommended by your dentist or dental hygienist.

- Use the oral care products recommended by your dental care professional. Some are used every day, while others are used for treating a specific problem. These include toothpastes, mouthwashes, toothbrushes, oral antiseptics, dental bleaching agents, and other products, such as floss and picks.

5

Body Fitness

Good eating habits and a fit body go hand-in-hand. Ideally, the number of calories you consume should match the number you burn. A certain number of calories are necessary for body functions and activities. This number depends on your body size, gender, and stage in life. When more calories are consumed than the body needs, the excess is stored as body fat. Each pound of excess body fat is produced from 3,500 calories. A combination of diet and exercise usually promote weight loss and improves body fitness. Once you are at your ideal weight, continued exercise will help you maintain it.

Determining How Weight Affects Health

The Body Mass Index (BMI) is an important tool to evaluate your weight and determine your risk of developing additional health problems. BMI is a common measure used to determine if you are overweight, obese, underweight, or normal. BMI takes into account a person's weight and height to gauge total body fat in adults. The higher the BMI is, the greater the risk of developing additional health problems. BMI *correlates* with body fat. The relationship between fatness and BMI differs with age and gender. For example, women are more likely to have a higher percentage of body fat than men for the same BMI. On average, older people may have more body fat than younger adults with the same BMI.

BMI equals a person's weight divided by height squared ($BMI=kg/m^2$ or lb/ft^2). It will, however, overestimate fatness in people who are muscular or athletic. Since BMI calculations use total body weight and not estimates of lean muscle mass and fat, it cannot determine between the overweight and the more muscular. BMI testing does not work for anyone under 18, for body-builders, or for pregnant or nursing women.

Women tend to believe they look their best at values between the range of 20 to 22 and men are usually satisfied with a BMI of 23 to 25. Generally, if your BMI falls within the range of 20 to 24.99, you are within the healthy weight range for your height and the risk of weight-related health problems is very small. Even though, a BMI under 20 may seem desirable, you may be at risk of underweight-related illness, such as disappearance of periods (women), bone loss, malnutrition, and other conditions.

If your BMI is 26 or more, your risk of health problems becomes higher. In a recent study, an increased rate of high blood pressure, diabetes, and heart disease was recorded at 27.3 for women and 27.8 for men. For any BMI 30 and over, you are considered obese. Physicians rate obesity in various classes with associated weight-related health problems. It is a good idea to schedule a visit with your doctor to discuss your overall health condition and find out the best way to reduce your weight and risk.

BMI Is Not the Only Indicator of Health Risk

BMI is just one of many factors related to developing a chronic disease (such as heart disease, cancer, or diabetes). Other factors that may be important to look at when assessing your risk for chronic disease include diet, physical activity, waist circumference, blood pressure, blood sugar level, cholesterol level, and family history of disease.

Measure Your Waist Circumference

Another tool used to evaluate weight is your waist circumference. This is an especially helpful tool for people who are classified as overweight based on their BMI. That extra bit of fat, your spare tire, around the waist, is also a pre-dictor of health problems. Having the information about waist circumference coupled with BMI gives extra insight into how serious a health problem over-weight really poses. It is better to be pear shaped rather than to have an apple-shaped silhouette. This is true even if your BMI shows you at a healthy weight.

To obtain a proper measurement, stand up and measure around your waist, just above your hipbones. The more your waist measurement increases, the greater your health risks. If you are a woman whose waist measures more than

35 inches or a man whose waist measures more than 40 inches, you may be at greater risk for health problems including diabetes, high blood fats, high blood pressure, and heart disease. This is true even if your BMI shows you at a healthy weight.

Impact of Your Weight on Your Overall Health

Look at your overall health; decide what impact your weight has and what you should work on to improve your health. If you have a BMI of 25 to 30 and waist circumference of greater than 35 (for women) or 40 or more (for men) *and* one or more risk factors, *or* your BMI is greater than 30 and you have one or more risk factors, then you need to talk to your doctor to see if you are at an increased risk for disease and if you should lose weight. Even a small weight loss (just 10% of your current weight) may help lower the risk of disease. A complete health assessment by a physician is the best way to decide the right steps for you.

The BMI will give you a baseline of your level of body fat and how much you should weigh. It's not the rule; it's just a guideline. It's unhealthy to have anxiety over a less-than-perfect body image. Physical activity and good nutrition are key factors in leading a healthy lifestyle and reducing risk for disease. You are taking steps to improve your health and fitness just by reading this book and becoming informed about health and fitness issues. Remember, a healthy mental attitude is just as important as physical fitness.

Calculating Your Body Mass Index

The BMI chart is an easy way to understand your body fitness. To find your Body Mass Index using the Body Mass Index Chart:

1. Find your height in inches, in the left-hand column.

2. Look across the row for your weight in pounds.

3. Then look up your BMI in the top column.

For example, you are 60 inches tall, and your weigh is 118 pounds. Then, your Body Mass Index is 23 (Normal weight). If you are 64 inches in height and your weight is 173 pounds. Then, your Body Mass Index is 30 (Obese).

BMI	19	20	21	22	23	24	25	26	27	28	29	30	31	32	33	34	35	36	37	38	39	40
Height											Weight in Pounds											
58"	91	96	100	105	110	115	119	124	129	134	138	143	148	153	158	162	167	172	177	181	186	191
59"	94	99	104	109	114	119	124	128	133	138	143	148	153	158	163	168	173	178	183	188	193	198
60"	97	102	107	112	118	123	128	133	138	143	148	153	158	163	168	174	179	184	189	194	199	204
61"	100	106	111	116	122	127	132	137	143	148	153	158	164	169	174	180	185	190	195	201	206	211
62"	104	109	115	120	126	131	136	142	147	153	158	164	169	175	181	186	191	196	202	207	213	218
63"	107	113	118	124	130	135	141	146	152	158	163	169	175	180	186	191	197	203	208	214	220	225
64"	110	116	122	128	134	140	145	151	157	163	169	174	180	186	192	197	204	209	215	221	227	232
65"	114	120	126	132	138	144	150	156	162	168	174	180	186	192	198	204	210	216	222	228	234	240
66"	118	124	130	136	142	148	155	161	167	173	179	186	192	198	204	210	216	223	229	235	241	247
67"	121	127	134	140	146	153	159	166	172	178	185	191	198	204	211	217	223	230	236	242	249	255
68"	125	131	138	144	151	158	164	171	177	184	190	197	203	210	216	223	230	236	243	249	256	262
69"	128	135	142	149	155	162	169	176	182	189	196	203	209	216	223	230	236	243	250	257	263	270
70"	132	139	146	153	160	167	174	181	188	195	202	209	216	222	229	236	243	250	257	264	271	278
71"	136	143	150	157	165	172	179	186	193	200	208	215	222	229	236	243	250	257	265	272	279	286
72"	140	147	154	162	169	177	184	191	199	206	213	221	228	235	242	250	258	265	272	279	287	294
73"	144	151	159	166	174	182	189	197	204	212	219	227	235	242	250	257	265	272	280	288	295	302
74"	148	155	163	171	179	186	194	202	210	218	225	233	241	249	256	264	272	280	287	295	303	311
75"	152	160	168	176	184	192	200	208	216	224	232	240	248	254	264	272	279	287	295	303	311	319
76"	156	164	172	180	189	197	205	213	221	230	238	246	254	263	271	279	287	295	304	312	320	328

You can also calculate your BMI yourself by using either of these formulas:

BMI = Weight (in pounds) × 704.5 divided by (Height [in inches] × Height [in inches])

BMI = Weight (in kilograms) divided by (Height [in meters] × Height [in meters])

- Divide your height in centimeters by 2.54 to convert it into inches. Multiply your weight in kilograms by 2.2 to convert it into pounds.

For example, you are 158 centimeters in height. The calculation is 158 divided by 2.54 centimeters equals 62 inches. Your weight is 77 kilograms. The calculation is 77 multiplied by 2.2 pounds equals 169 pounds. Then, your Body Mass Index is 31 (Obese).

An Overall Body Fitness Plan

Fitness leads to an improved sense of well-being, improved appearance, enhanced social life, and increased stamina and strength. It also reduces your risk of developing chronic diseases, such as high blood pressure, hardening of the arteries, and diabetes.

Most experts agree that overall fitness consists of three areas:

- **Flexibility:** The ability to move joints and use muscles through their full range of motion. Stretching is a flexibility exercise.

- **Aerobic fitness:** The conditioning of your heart and lungs. It increases the amount of oxygen that is delivered to your muscles, which allows them to work longer. Walking is a type of aerobic exercise.

- **Strengthening:** Muscle strengthening includes building more powerful muscles and increasing how long you can use them (endurance). Weight lifting builds stronger muscles and strengthens bones, while push-ups build endurance.

Before starting any fitness or exercise program, consult your doctor for a complete checkup. Exercising should not hurt. Exercising may cause minor soreness only. If more discomfort is felt during exercise, stop immediately and consult your doctor.

Flexibility Fitness

Stretching elongates your muscles, which keeps them flexible. Stretching helps you avoid muscle aches and pains that may result from your aerobic and strength fitness programs. It also increases your balance and stability, enhances blood circulation, and helps relaxation. Stretching before and after aerobic exercise (even walking) and muscle strengthening help you feel better and may help you avoid injury.

For extensive flexibility fitness, you may want to participate in activities that include stretching, such as dance, martial arts (aikido or karate), tai chi, or yoga. There is a set of flexibility exercises in Appendix A.

Aerobic Fitness

Aerobic fitness burns fat and calories, and allows muscles to work at a steady rate with a constant supply of oxygen-rich blood. Your body's nourishment occurs at a faster pace. You shave off extra weight, your muscle tone is improved, your blood pressure goes down, you decrease your risk of heart disease, stress is reduced, your energy increases, and your mood improves. That's naming just a few of the benefits. All in addition to getting that healthy-looking glow! Here are a variety of aerobic activities that you may include in your 20- to 30-minute aerobic fitness activity: brisk walking (outdoors or on a treadmill), running (outdoors or on a treadmill), biking (stationary or outdoor), jogging in place, swimming, skating, rowing, hiking, jumping rope, race-walking, stair climbing, bench stepping, cross-country skiing (outdoor or skiing machine), using the elliptical trainer, engaging in low-impact aerobics and dancing.

Easy Aerobic Fitness, Walk More!

You can easily add aerobic fitness into your daily routine just by adding walking or walking more. Here are a few ways:

- Park your car in a parking spot at the far end of the lot, whether it's near work, the supermarket, the mall, or the cinema.

- If you take public transportation (bus, cab, subway, streetcar), get off ten blocks before your destination and walk the remainder of the way.

- Sign up for a weekly charity walk.

- Volunteer to walk dogs at an animal shelter or walk your own dog daily.

- In rainy or snowy weather, walk briskly around a mall for 20 or more minutes.

- Take the stairs instead of the elevator.

- Walk around the block several times while you wait for your child to take a music lesson.

- Walk around medical buildings if you have a long wait for a doctor's appointment. Ask the receptionist to give you an idea of how long your wait will be.

- If you dine out at lunch, walk to a nearby restaurant.

- If you have a meeting in another nearby building, leave 5 or 10 minutes early and walk to the building. Walk back to your building after the meeting.

- Walk to work, if you live near by.

- Walk to your shopping center if it is near where you live or work.

Remember to start your aerobic fitness program with flexibility exercises. Then, complete your aerobic fitness with flexibility exercises to cool down your muscles and help prevent aches and pains.

Strength Fitness

Strength fitness builds muscle. As you build muscle, you will lose fat. Muscles burn more calories than fat. When your body is at rest, strength fitness can actually speed up your metabolism! You can eat more healthful food without gaining weight or you can lose weight more quickly if you need to. Current research also shows that strength fitness helps keep bones strong, helping to prevent osteoporosis or bone loss that concerns many women after menopause.

Strength training using weights can be done at a health club, a community or fitness center that has a weight room, with home equipment, or at a weight room in your apartment complex or community. You may use free weights (barbells and dumbbells), resistance-training machines (weights attached to cables and pulleys), or your own body weight (calisthenics). The benefit of going to a health club or center is that they provide professional training on the proper exercise form, which helps prevent injuries and which you can use both at the club and on your home equipment. Knowing the proper techniques can help you get the most out of your strength training.

Push-ups, crunches, lunges, and squats are also strengthening exercises. You only need to do strength fitness two or three times a week, and you need to rest at least a day in between to allow time for your muscles to heal, recover, and strengthen between workouts. It is a good idea to alternate your aerobic fitness with strength fitness. Swimming, cycling, and skiing are activities that improve both muscle strength and aerobic fitness. There is a set of strengthening exercises in Appendix A.

Weekly Overall Fitness Program

To achieve fitness, most experts recommend either of the following:

- Moderate activity for 30 minutes a day, 5 days a week or more. Moderate activity is activity equal to a brisk walk.

- Vigorous exercise for 20 minutes a day, 3 times a week or more. Vigorous activity is activity that provides 70 percent or more of your maximum heart rate. The heart rate is how many times your heart beats in a minute. The maximum heart rate is the fastest the heart can beat at your maximum activity level. The maximum heart rate changes as you age. A percentage of the maximum heart rate is often used to determine the intensity of exercise.

An easier way to determine if your heart rate is above 70 percent of your maximum heart rate is perceived exertion. This is a subjective measure of how hard you're working based primarily on your breathing. The scale goes from zero to ten, with level zero being how it feels to be at rest and level ten being an exertion so difficult you could probably only maintain it for a few seconds. Being at 70 percent of your maximum heart rate is about a level seven or eight. At level seven, you feel fatigue but are certain that you can maintain the pace for the rest of your session. Your breathing is deep, but you can still carry on a conversation. Level eight is slightly more vigorous; you may be able to still carry on a conversation, but you wouldn't want to.

Alternate your Aerobic Fitness with Strength Fitness during the week. You should plan on taking one day off for rest. Wear comfortable clothing, such as loose-fitting shorts or elasticized-waist knit lounge pants, a T-shirt, and athletic shoes. If you walk during your lunch hour at your workplace, you may just want to wear your normal work clothing; just make sure you are comfortable in it, and wear comfortable shoes.

Aerobic Fitness Day: Burn Fat/Cardiovascular Health
Flexibility Fitness: 5 minutes
Aerobic Fitness: 20–30 minutes
Flexibility Fitness: 5 minutes

Strength Fitness Day: Build Muscle/Tone Body
Flexibility Fitness: 5 minutes
Strength Fitness: 20–30 minutes
Flexibility Fitness: 5 minutes

Fitness Activities and Calories Burned

Here is a chart of fitness activities ranging from mild-to-moderate to moderate-to-intense exercise and the approximate number of calories that a 150-pound person may burn over one hour's time. The calories spent in a particular activity vary in proportion to your body weight. If you are 100 pounds, you burn one-third fewer calories than a 150-pound person, so multiply the number of calories burned per hour in the chart by one-third. If you are 200 pounds, you burn one-third more calories than a 150-pound person, so multiply the number of calories burned per hour in the chart by two-thirds.

Fitness Activities and Calories Burned

Mild-to-Moderate	Calories Burned Per Hour
Tennis	425
Bicycling or stationary cycling (10 mph)	415
Hiking with a 20-pound backpack (3 mph)	400
Aerobics, moderate intensity	350
Horseback riding	350
Inline or roller skating	350
Square dancing	350
Treadmill walking (4 mph)	345
Gardening	323
Tennis (doubles)	312
Ballroom dancing	300
Calisthenics	300
Rowing machine, low intensity	300
Strength training	300
Table tennis	300
Aerobics, low impact	275
Golf, walking with clubs	270
Volleyball	264
Bicycling or stationary cycling (5.5 mph)	245
Walking, mild (2 to 2.5 mph)	185 to 255
Light housework, cleaning	246
Canoeing (2.5 mph)	174

Fitness Activities and Calories Burned

Moderate-to-Intense	Calories Burned Per Hour
Marital Arts	790
Circuit weight training	756
Running (7.2 mph)	700
Stair-climbing machine	680
Rope-jumping	660
Bicycling or stationary cycling (13 mph)	655
Rowing machine, moderate intensity	655
Running/jogging (5.5 mph)	655
Step aerobics, moderate intensity	610
Cross-country skiing (5 mph)	600
Handball	600
Racquetball	588
Walking, vigorous (5 mph)	555
Polka dancing, without the beer	540
Swimming	540
Football (touch, vigorous)	498
Basketball	450
Tennis (singles)	450
Ice skating (9 mph)	384
Inline skating (9 mph)	384

Mystery Weight Gains

Body Weight Fluctuates Daily

This fluctuation is due to changes in the body fluids that make up approximately 70 percent of our total body weight. Hormonal changes, the amount of carbohydrates and salt in your diet, and exercise affect these fluids. Weigh yourself at regular intervals during the month, but not every day! Weight changes over several weeks will reflect changes in levels of fat and muscle, rather than body fluid. Avoid fluid retention by avoiding salty and highly seasoned foods and lightly salting your food. Eat a sufficient quantity of potassium-rich vegetables and fruits because potassium offsets sodium, thus reducing fluid retention. This fluid retention can explain why you may gain a pound or two after dining out and eating highly seasoned food.

Stress Hormone Influences Weight Gain

Cortisol is one of several hormones made in the adrenal glands. It is important for normal carbohydrate metabolism and response to stress. Cortisol is also known as the "stress hormone." The primary responsibility of cortisol is to activate the immune system; it also is involved with the metabolism of glucose and can cause elevation of the blood sugar level. Cortisol has many actions in the body, and one ultimate goal of cortisol secretion is to provide energy.

Cortisol stimulates fat and carbohydrate metabolism for fast energy, and stimulates insulin release and maintenance of blood sugar levels. The end result of these actions is an increase in appetite. Thus chronic stress, or poorly managed stress, may lead to cortisol levels that stimulate your appetite, with the end result being weight gain or difficulty losing unwanted pounds. Cortisol not only promotes weight gain, but it can also affect where you put on the weight. Doctors have shown that stress and elevated cortisol tend to cause fat deposition in the abdominal area rather than in the hips. This fat deposition has been referred to as "toxic fat" since abdominal fat deposition is strongly correlated with the development of cardiovascular disease including heart attacks and strokes.

Whether your stress levels will result in high cortisol levels and weight gain is not readily predictable. The amount of cortisol secreted in response to stress can vary among individuals, with some persons being innately more "reactive" to stressful events.

Experts agree that stress management is a critical part of weight loss regimens, particularly in those who have elevated cortisol levels. Exercise is the best and fastest method for weight loss in this case, since exercise leads to the release of endorphins, which have natural stress-fighting properties and can lower cortisol levels. Activities such as yoga and meditation can also help lower stress hormone levels. To effectively reduce elevated cortisol due to stress, lifestyle changes are essential.

Begin recognizing and managing your stress by:

- **Developing relaxation skills.** Several relaxation techniques are discussed in Chapter 6.

- **Paying attention to physical health.** Stress results from a combination of physical and mental factors. If your body isn't able to handle these challenges, you aren't going to be capable of effectively managing your stress level.

- **Exercising regularly.** Exercise not only stimulates the release of endorphins, the body's natural stress-fighters, but it also helps lower cortisol and other stress hormone levels.

- **Prioritizing commitments and responsibilities.** Learn to differentiate between mandatory obligations and commitments you've made due to guilt, to satisfy others, or to fulfill unrealistic expectations of yourself. Learning to say no can help you reduce the stress of excessive demands on your time and energy. If your stress is job-related, it is time to think about whether that job is worth the poor health, physical and mental. This may be your body's way to telling you to move on to a different job or line of work.

- **Getting more sleep.** Poor sleep and stressful days can evolve into a vicious cycle. The inability to sleep may actually make some of us more prone to stress. Doctors have shown that levels of cortisol were higher in people with chronic insomnia and suggested that people with insomnia might have a hyperactive body response to stress. Ways to enhance your sleep are discussed in Chapter 6.

- **Reducing caffeine.** Caffeine raises the production of cortisol. Studies have shown that as little as two to three cups of coffee can raise your cortisol level. Heavy coffee consumption can lead to a state of adrenal gland exhaustion, where the adrenal glands are no longer able to respond adequately to stress by releasing enough adrenaline. Adrenal insufficiency can then lead to a host of other problems, including a weakened immune response, anxiety, and panic attacks. Caffeine also interferes with adenosine, a brain chemical that normally has a calming effect, and raises the level of lactate, a biochemical known to produce panic attacks. Switching to tea, therefore reducing your caffeine intake, can sometimes make all the difference.

Food Intolerance, Allergies, or Sensitivities

Intolerance to a certain food can give many of the signs and symptoms of stress. It is widely believed that stress itself can result in intolerance to a variety of foods and a few overweight people may show increased hypersensitivity to foods. These sensitivities can result in a reduced ability to metabolize fats. Allergic symptoms often develop from overexposure to the same food over a long period. The difference between food allergy and food intolerance is that a food allergy, or hypersensitivity, is an abnormal response to a food that is triggered by the immune system; with food intolerance, the immune system is not responsible for the symptoms, even though they may resemble those of a food allergy.

Food intolerance can trigger responses that cause bloating or fluid retention. When the body detects an allergen, it releases histamines and other chemicals to the affected areas, which swell up in response. As we age, our production of digestive enzymes diminishes, creating a greater chance of developing allergic reactions to foods. You can be allergic to any food, but there are certain foods that seem to have a higher allergy factor than others. The two most common food allergens are wheat and dairy. Other food allergens are rye, corn, eggs, beef, fish and shellfish, nuts, chocolate, sugar, coffee, tea, tomatoes, alcohol (red and port wine), yeast, all preservatives and colorings, and mold that grows on food or is part of its creation, such as cheese, wine, beer, and mushrooms. In addition, many medications used to treat allergy symptoms often trigger weight gain as a side effect, without ever addressing the actual cause of the immune response.

A doctor can perform tests to distinguish a food allergy from food intolerance. Common food intolerances that mimic food allergies include:

- Dairy or lactose intolerance

- Reaction to preservatives, flavorings, and colorings, such as monosodium glutamate (MSG) and sulfites (added to foods to provide crispness and part of the fermentation of wine)

- Wheat sensitivity and gluten intolerance

- Sugar sensitivity

- Yeast sensitivity

Hormonal Changes in Women

Women in their forties and fifties will notice that with hormonal changes during this time in their lives, body fat will tend to be redistributed from the thighs, buttocks, and hips to the breast and stomach areas. After menopause, the body does not burn the substantial amount of calories it did during the first two weeks of each menstrual cycle during the process of ovulation. The extra calories that the body used to use may now be stored as stomach fat. Also, be aware of the weight creep from too many alcoholic beverages. During this phase of life, be wary of getting a little too sedentary; with hormonal changes and a few extra drinks, the calories may not be burned as efficiently as they were before. Additionally, this weight gain is accompanied by increases in blood sugar and insulin, which can put a person at risk of heart disease.

So, body toning becomes ever so important. By being physically active, your body puts on muscle, which will raise your metabolism, because muscle tissue burns off calories, even while at rest. Continue eating wisely and continue daily physical activity and strength training.

The Skin You're In

As we age, our skin inevitably changes. Some of the signs of aging skin are dryness and dullness, rough texture, lines and wrinkles, uneven tone, and age spots. Long-term, inadequate nutrition can also lead to these changes. Some researchers suggest that crinkled, crepe-like skin is the result of inflammation. However, it's never too late to improve its condition with inner and outer care.

First, Nourish Your Skin from the Inside

Eating a diet high in antioxidant and anti-inflammatory vegetables and fruits will help maintain healthy skin. These are the deep green and brightly colored ones. Their antioxidant vitamins and phytochemicals neutralize the free radicals. The more antioxidants your body has, the more protection they can provide.

Eat enough complete protein (protein that has all the essential amino acids—animal protein). We are made of protein: our muscles, skin, bones, internal organs, antibodies, and enzymes. Protein is essential to regenerate and repair cells. Without adequate protein, our bodies' cell repair process slows and can be incomplete, resulting in a breakdown of cells and interfering with our body's ability to repair them.

Keeping hydrated by drinking a minimum of eight 8-ounces glasses of water daily nourishes your skin from the inside. Healthy, hydrated cells are plump, whereas dehydrated cells sag. Dry skin is more prone to wrinkling, cracking, eczema, irritation, and flaking. Drinking green tea in addition to your daily intake of water is also beneficial. Green tea's phytochemicals, called catechins, have significant anticancer and antibacterial effects.

Don't forget why you are ingesting olive oil and flaxseed oil, nuts and seeds. They provide essential anti-inflammatory and antioxidant protection. Current research links fewer skin wrinkles to an increase in omega-3 fatty acids, so take that flaxseed!

Additionally, smoking deprives skin tissue of oxygen and nutrients through the effects of carbon monoxide and nicotine in the circulatory system, giving a pale complexion and early wrinkles. Caffeine and alcohol dehydrate the skin, the latter being even more damaging by impeding circulation, removing moisture and nutrients, and even leading to broken or distended capillaries.

Second, Nourish Your Skin from the Outside

This is about your overall body skin care. Sometimes, we neglect the rest of us, since we usually present our best face. We pay more attention to our feet during the summer months when we wear open-toed shoes. When do we pay attention to our ears? Practicing good overall skin care on the outside is the polish to the apple of you! Here are a few basics:

- **Cleanse:** Start with clean skin. Cleansing is critical to healthy skin. Removing the skin's natural oils along with dirt and environmental pollution is the first requirement in creating healthier skin.

- **Exfoliate:** Slough off dead, flaking skin and rough spots. The average skin cell life is about thirty days. Use a gentle exfoliating scrub or gently rub your body with a loofah or body brush. The key word here is *gentle,* not harsh scrubbing; you don't want to abrade your skin! You'll want to exfoliate your skin no more than once a week, or twice a month if your skin is sensitive.

- **Moisturize:** Moisturizing will protect your skin, lock in moisture, and provide a healthy supply of essential nutrients daily. Use topical creams and lotions that provide moisturizing, antioxidant protection, anti-inflammatory protection, and aid in skin regeneration.

  This includes a basic all-around moisturizer and two types of body lotions: one that has alpha hydroxy acid or glycolic acid and the other that contains vitamin C ester. Use a lotion daily, alternating type every other day. Apply the moisturizer all over your body skin, including your ears and feet. Massage gently into hands and body. Moisturizers tend to be most effective after a bath or shower when skin is slightly wet.

- **Sunscreen:** Protect your skin from overexposure to the sun year-round. When you plan on being in the sun longer than twenty minutes, apply a broad-spectrum sunscreen with both ultraviolet A and B (UVA and UVB) ray protection and an SPF of at least 15.

- Avoid sun exposure when sun is at its strongest, between 10:00 A.M. and 3:00 P.M.

- Wear protective clothing in harsh environments, such as long sleeves, pants, and hats.

- Reduce exposure to environmental pollution.

- Visit your doctor for regular skin cancer screenings.

Use a Basic Moisturizer

The most important thing to remember about moisturizers is that a good moisturizing product can improve the texture of your skin by protecting it. There are four basic classes of body moisturizers: ointments, oils, creams, and lotions (listed in decreasing order of moisturizing power).

- **Ointment moisturizers:** These products have the greatest ability to trap moisture in the skin, but they have the greasy consistency and feel of Vaseline Petroleum Jelly. To minimize the greasy feel, apply a small amount and rub it into the skin well (when the skin takes on a sheen). Examples of effective ointment moisturizers include Aquaphor and plain Vaseline Petroleum Jelly. In addition to brand-name moisturizers, some common household products, such as vegetable shortening, can be used as very inexpensive body moisturizers. Again, the key to using an ointment is to apply small amounts and rub it in well.

- **Oil moisturizers:** These products are less greasy but still effective. Oils that can be applied directly to the skin include baby oil, mineral oil, vegetable oil, and bath oil. Bath oils used in the bath water make the tub too slippery and should not be used. It is preferable to apply bath oils after getting out of the tub or shower, just as you would moisturizers, directly to partially dry skin.

- **Cream moisturizers:** These are usually white and disappear when rubbed into the skin without leaving a greasy feel. As a result they tend to be more popular than ointments. Examples of effective cream moisturizers include Original Eucerin Cream, Cetaphil Moisturizing Cream, Vaseline Cream,

Nutraderm, Nivea, and Neutrogena Hand Cream-Norwegian Formula (especially helpful for dry, chapped hands and cuticles).

• **Lotion moisturizers:** These are suspensions of oily chemicals in alcohol and water. Lotion moisturizers are generally the least greasy and the most pleasant to use and therefore are quite popular. However, because of their alcohol content, they can be somewhat drying when used repeatedly compared to ointments and creams. The bottom line is that if the moisturizer you choose does not feel at least a bit greasy, you may not be getting as strong a moisturizer as you might need. Examples of popular lotion moisturizers include Vaseline Intensive Care, Nutraderm, Keri, Lubriderm, Curel, Nivea, Neutrogena, Moisturel, and Lac-Hydrin 5.

Use an Alpha Hydroxy Acid Body Lotion

Alpha hydroxy acids (AHA) are organic acids that are popular in cosmetic preparations because of their beneficial effects on the appearance of skin. Gylcolic acid is one form of AHA that is derived from fruit. A benefit of glycolic acid is that it improves dry, thickened, sun-damaged, and problem-prone skin. However, exactly how glycolic acid improves the skin's appearance is still not known. It is thought to work through a combination of reducing inflammation, promoting earlier removal of dry skin scales, and optimizing moisturization, which results in a more normal looking, healthy epidermis. AHA products cause exfoliation, or shedding of the surface skin. The extent of exfoliation depends on the type and concentration of the AHA, its pH (acidity), and other ingredients in the product. AHA products may increase your skin's sensitivity to the sun and particularly the possibility of sunburn. Limit sun exposure while using an AHA product and use a sunscreen for a week afterward.

Some products will contain beta hydroxy acid (BHA) or salicylic acid, which appears to be less irritating than alpha hydroxy acid. This is because salicylic acid is derived from acetylsalicylic acid, or aspirin. Aspirin has anti-inflammatory properties, and salicylic acid retains many of these anti-inflammatory properties.

When selecting an AHA body lotion, read the product label to make sure that the AHA is one of the first ten ingredients in the product. Manufacturers must list the ingredients on the package in the order of their concentration in the product. When comparing products with AHAs, if one product has an

AHA listed as the second item and another product has an AHA listed as the fifth ingredient, then the first product has more of the AHA ingredient than the second product. Some AHA products will list the AHA concentration on the package. Choose an AHA concentration of 10 percent or less, with a pH of 3.5 (acidity) or greater, and one that is formulated to protect the skin from increased sun sensitivity.

Examples of AHA body lotions include Vaseline Intensive Care Healthy Body Complexion (lactic acid/lactates are the AHAs), Neutrogena Skin Smoothing Body Lotion (sodium glycolate/salicylic acid are the AHA/BHA), Jergens Skin Smoothing Moisturizer (lactic acid/tridecyl salicylate are the AHA/BHA), and Walgreens Alpha Hydroxy Lotion with 8% AHA (glycolic acid is the AHA). These products can be found in most supermarkets and drugstores. Store brands (such as Walgreens) that have the same list of ingredients as those listed can be just as effective at a lower cost.

Use a Vitamin C Ester Body Lotion

The benefits of this new skin care discovery have profound benefits. The antioxidant properties of vitamin C ester protect against free radicals that can have a cumulative damage effect on skin. Those occur from environmental pollutants, sun overexposure, and general skin metabolism.

Vitamin C ester (ascorbyl palmitate) boosts protective antioxidant action, is fat-soluble, which aids in penetrating the skin, and helps repair past damage by aiding new collagen production. It is a scientifically advanced form of vitamin C (created by adding a fatty acid from palm oil), with solubility that allows absorption to take place more easily than other forms of vitamin C and with less irritation. Some of these vitamin C ester formulations use magnesium ascorbyl phosphate. Examples of vitamin C body lotions include Jergens Replenishing Multi-Vitamin A, E & C, Revlon Vitamin C Absolute Re-Energizing Body Lotion, Avalon Organics Vitamin C Therapeutic Hand and Body Lotion, and Jason Hand and Body Lotion Vitamins A, C & E. The Jergens and Revlon brands can be found at most supermarkets and drugstores. The others can be found in natural-food stores.

6

Relax; Take It Easy

There's much evidence that relaxation techniques can have a positive effect on the immune response and resilience to disease. Learning ways to relax can have many benefits, perhaps the most important of which is developing a feeling of confidence about facing the everyday challenges of life, including:

- Reducing unhealthy stress and anxiety
- Increasing resistance to illness and disease
- Lowering blood pressure
- Reducing the heart rate
- Relieving muscle tension
- Coping with medical problems, such as chronic pain or diabetes
- Preventing, managing, and coping with migraine headaches
- Coping with extremely stressful or painful situations

While a certain amount of stress can be beneficial, stimulating the body and mind to improve your performance, too much stress causes over-stimulation and leads to physical and mental illnesses. *Stress management* refers to a strategy of controlling stress and reducing its impact. Adopting appropriate coping mechanisms can relieve stress in a healthy, productive way. Stress management includes all aspects of your life: physical, emotional, and behavioral well-being, nutrition, exercise, the amount of sleep you get, leisure activities, coping skills, communication skills, and relationship management. Stress management techniques also include meditation, yoga, and relaxation techniques. Many health centers and hospitals either offer classes in such techniques or can refer you to classes at other locations.

Easy Relaxation Techniques

When used consistently, relaxation techniques can prove effective in controlling stress by helping you reach a state of mental calm, even when you are in the middle of a stressful situation. Here are a few easy relaxation techniques you can practice to prevent or ease stress-induced illness.

The Relaxation Response

The Relaxation Response is a simple technique that can relieve stress and tension. It was developed by Herbert Benson, M.D., at Harvard Medical School. He conducted extensive testing and included the results in his book, *The Relaxation Response.*

- Select fifteen minutes in your day, preferably early evening, before dinner when you'll be free of distractions. If you prefer to relax later in the evening, do so two hours after any meal, since the digestive processes seem to interfere with the elicitation of the relaxation response. Keep a watch or clock nearby so you can check your time periodically.

- Choose a focus word or short phrase that has some resonance for you. No, it does not need to be "Ohm"; it could be "Jumping Jack Flash." Just pick a word or words that are calming to you.

- Sitting quietly in a comfortable position in a comfortable chair, and close your eyes. Breathe slowly and normally, repeating the word silently as you exhale.

- Consciously relax your muscles, beginning from your toes, moving up to your feet, then ankles, calves, knees, thighs, hips, stomach, chest, shoulders, upper arms, elbows, lower arms, wrists, hands, fingers, then your neck, and finally, your head.

- Keep breathing evenly and keep repeating your word or phrase. Sometimes, other thoughts will come whirling in like a hamster running in its exercise wheel. Acknowledge these thoughts, and let them move through you; you can address them after you finish.

- When fifteen minutes have elapsed, sit quietly for a few minutes with your eyes still closed, and then open them.

- You will most likely be in a more peaceful and a calmer state. This state is your body's natural relaxation response. See, easy, without any fancy mediation techniques to learn.

Breath Counting

Breath counting is another simple relaxation technique that takes ten minutes.

- Select ten minutes in your day when you'll be free of distractions. Keep a watch or clock nearby so you can check your time periodically.

- Sit quietly in a comfortable position in a comfortable chair, and close your eyes. Take a few deep breaths. Then breathe naturally. It should be quiet and slow.

- Count 1 to yourself as you exhale.

- Upon the next exhaled breath, count 2. Continue counting your exhaled breath up to 5.

- Begin a new cycle of counting five breaths. Sometimes, your mind will wander and you may find yourself counting more than five breaths. That's okay; just go back and start at 1 again.

- When ten minutes have elapsed, sit quietly for a few minutes with your eyes still closed, and then open them.

Visualization or Guided Imagery

In addition to reducing stress, visualization can direct the stress to create a more positive mental performance. Many athletes use visualization during training.

- Select ten minutes in your day when you'll be free of distractions. Keep a watch or clock nearby so you can check your time periodically.

- Sit quietly in a comfortable position in a comfortable chair, and close your eyes. Take a few deep breaths. Then breathe naturally. It should be quiet and slow.

- Imagine a relaxing scene. If you enjoy relaxing at the beach, imagine a beach scene. If you prefer a garden, then imagine a garden scene.

Imagine all the details of the scene with vibrant colors, sounds, aromas, tastes, textures, and emotion. For example, if you find the beach a place of relaxation, perhaps you'd see the blue water and sky, white sand and caps of the waves, and green palm trees. You'd likely hear the waves, the seagulls, and the wind. You'd smell fish and taste the salt in the air. You'd feel the smoothness and the wetness of the water and the grittiness of the sand. You'd likely experience a sense of peace and serenity. The use of visualization can take you on a trip for little effort and without any expense.

- When your mind wanders, bring it firmly back to your scene. Concentrate on the image and make every effort to exclude everything else. This may be difficult at first, but will become easier with practice.

- When ten minutes have elapsed, sit quietly for a few minutes with your eyes still closed, and then open them.

Using Visualization for Stress at Work

If you know that you have a stressful meeting, a confrontation, or a social situation coming up, you can prepare yourself by using visualization.

- Select ten minutes when you'll be free of distractions. Keep a watch or clock nearby so you can check your time periodically.

- Sit quietly in a comfortable position in a comfortable chair, and close your eyes. Take a few deep breaths. Then breathe naturally. It should be quiet and slow.

- Imagine the meeting, confrontation, or social situation—the location, the people present, and agendas at hand.

- Rehearse the various scenes in your mind; picture what will produce the stress, however small the detail is.

- Distance yourself from the problem and relax, breathing deeply and evenly. At first, you may find that tension arises, but as you continue the tension will ease away.

- Once you have confronted and overcome one problem, go to the next one.

- When ten minutes have elapsed, sit quietly for a few minutes with your eyes still closed, and then open them.

- By the time the meeting, confrontation, or social situation occurs, you will have reduced the stress it would have caused to a very manageable level or to no stress at all.

Autogenic Training

This relaxation technique is similar to visualization in that it works through self-suggestion but focuses on specific muscle relaxation. It can be helpful in reducing nervous tension, such as performance anxiety before an exam. This technique is popular in Europe and has been gaining increased acceptance in the United States and in other countries.

- Select fifteen minutes when you'll be free of distractions. Keep a watch or clock nearby so you can check your time periodically.

- Sit quietly in a comfortable position in a comfortable chair, and close your eyes. Take a few deep breaths. Then breathe naturally. It should be quiet and slow.

- Basic training starts with six simple phrases that must be practiced repeatedly in sequence. At the advanced level, additional suggestions may be incorporated into the training program. The six phrases are as follows:

  - My body is very heavy (promotes muscle relaxation).

  - I am very warm (relaxes your blood vessels and enhances circulation).

  - My heartbeat is calm and regular (regulates your pulse).

  - My breathing is calm and regular (relaxes your lungs and airways).

  - My abdomen is warm and relaxed (relaxes your stomach and exercises the abdominal wall).

  - My forehead is cool and clear (relieves tension in your head).

- Repeat the phrases and before the end of your relaxation period, add in a phrase that relates to your ailment, such as "my head is cool and clear" if you have a headache.

- When fifteen minutes have elapsed, sit quietly for a few minutes with your eyes still closed, and then open them.

Passive Relaxation Through Therapeutic Massage

Being massaged is another method to combat the symptoms of stress. Massage therapists work directly on the muscles and ligaments of the body. The massage relieves muscle tension and improves circulation and lymph drainage, thus helping the body rid itself of toxins. Its effect on the nervous system to calm, soothe, and give an overall sense of well-being is an ideal relaxation technique for busy people. There are various massage techniques, including sports, deep tissue, neuromuscular, Swedish, and Oriental.

Mindful Meditation

There are many types of meditation that you can practice to relax the mind and trigger the body's natural relaxation response. Many forms of meditation, such as Transcendental Meditation, require a teacher. However, mindfulness has been defined as the state of attention and awareness of present experiences, bringing yourself in touch with inner wisdom and to a moment-by-moment awareness of what you experience and feel. Paying attention to sounds, breathing rhythms, inner feelings, and your reaction patterns to specific situations are all part of being mindful. You can meditate mindfully by following these simple steps.

- Select fifteen minutes in your day when you'll be free of distractions. Keep a watch or clock nearby so you can check your time periodically.

- Sit quietly in a comfortable position in a comfortable chair, and close your eyes. Take a few deep breaths. Then breathe naturally. It should be quiet and slow.

- Gently notice your breathing. Refrain from trying to control or alter it in any way.

- Notice how your breath changes on its own accord. It may vary in speed, rhythm, or depth, and there may even be occasions when your breath seems to stop for a time. Whatever happens with your breathing, observe it without trying to cause any changes.

- Keep your focus on your breathing for the entire period.

- When fifteen minutes have elapsed, sit quietly for a few minutes with your eyes still closed, and then open them.

Enhancing Your Sleep

Sleep allows the body to complete its normal regenerative and restorative processes while the mind is at rest and not consciously in control of everything. Sleep is a natural body function during which we are relatively unconscious and the muscles that we normally control are relaxed. The result of sleep is refreshment of the nervous system (including the brain) and of the muscles. As we age, our bodies normally require less sleep. There are many medical expert opinions on how much sleep a person needs per night. Is it really the eight hours per night? Maybe or maybe not. Our sleep requirements are partly genetic; some of us need more, or less, than others. It ranges from five hours up to eleven hours a night.

Perhaps it is the *quality* of sleep that you get, rather than the *quantity* that makes all the difference in how refreshed you feel in the morning. Relaxation of the body and mind is key to enhancing the quality of your sleep and may increase the quantity over time.

Here are some techniques that may help you get started into a good night's rest. A few are relaxation techniques, some are nutritional, some are lifestyle changes, and some are environmental. Some of these techniques help when you have trouble falling asleep initially (taking more than thirty minutes to fall asleep) and some of them may help when you awaken in the middle of the night and have trouble getting back to sleep.

Nutritional

- **Drink warm milk.** A glass of warm milk fifteen minutes before going to bed will soothe your nervous system. Milk contains calcium, which works directly on jagged nerves to make them (and you) relax.

- **Eat a bedtime snack.** A snack that is relatively high in protein and low in carbohydrates is ideal, such as cheese, lean meat, or a piece of fruit. Also, hunger makes sleep difficult.

- **Avoid caffeine, alcohol, and tobacco.** The caffeine in coffee, nonherbal tea, and hot chocolate can disrupt sleep at night. Alcohol is a sedative, but it also disrupts the sleep mechanism, meaning that you are more apt to awaken in the middle of the night.

Environmental

- **Listen to soft, soothing music.** If you use silence to quiet your mind for a good night's rest, it often creates a need for the brain to make its own noise in the form of anxious thoughts. A good background for quiet is soft music, or nature sounds, particularly the sound of rain or the ocean.

- **Sleep in a well-ventilated room.** Fresh air and a room temperature between 60 and 65 degrees will give you the best sleeping conditions.

- **Sleep on a good firm bed.** It will give your entire body the support it needs to really relax.

- **Sleep in a dark room.** Any light source, even an illuminated bedroom clock, can be extremely annoying if you're having a hard time getting to sleep. If you can't block the light source, wear one of those eye pillows that the movie stars and international airline passengers wear.

Lifestyle Changes

- **Get some physical exercise during the day.** Regular exercise improves your ability to sleep well. Avoid vigorous exercise late in the evening; the hour or two before bedtime should be spent unwinding.

- **Keep regular bedtime hours.** The appropriate time to go to bed varies from individual to individual. We should normally go to bed only when we are tired and try to get up at a regular time each morning.

- **If you can't sleep, get up.** Don't lie awake trying to get to sleep any longer than thirty minutes. Get up. Do something quiet and non-stimulating. When you feel tired again, go back to bed

- **Don't watch TV or read before going to bed.** Wait at least one-half hour (preferably longer) before going to bed after reading or watching television. An over-stimulated mind, along with anxiety and stress, is what keeps you awake. It's all those thoughts in your head you have to get rid of before you can get to sleep.

- **Set aside a "worry" time.** Set a time earlier in the day to worry, plan, and make to-do lists.

Relaxation

- **Take a warm bath just before you go to bed.** Bathing will elevate your body temperature, and lying down will cause it to drop because your muscles will relax. Sleep tends to follow a decline in body temperature.

- **Practice relaxation techniques.**

Search for Body Sensations

- Lie on your back. Focus on your exhalation; exhale and relax.

- For two or three exhalations, focus on how your body feels on your bed.

- Following these exhalations, allow your attention to wander through your body. There is no set sequence and you should not be in a hurry. As you "move" through your body, identify any sensations that you may feel or sense (heaviness, warmth, heartbeat, coolness, twitching, pressure, gurgling in the stomach or intestines, tension, stillness.)

- Upon identifying a sensation, acknowledge the sensation in your mind's eye and continue to wander through the body and passively search for others. You will notice that the number of sensations diminishes after a few minutes. As the mind continues to focus inward on the body, the mind will become quiet and sleep will result.

Progressive Relaxation

- Lie on your back and close your eyes.

- Feel your feet. Feel the weight of your feet. Feel your feet relax and sink into the bed.

- Feel your lower legs. Feel the weight of your lower legs. Feel your lower legs relax and sink into the bed.

- Feel your knees. Feel the weight of your knees. Feel your knees relax and sink into the bed.

- Feel your upper legs. Feel the weight of your upper legs. Feel your upper legs relax and sink into the bed.

- Feel your hands. Feel the weight of your hands. Feel your hands relax and sink into the bed.

- Continue in this manner with your lower arms, elbows, upper arms, buttocks, back, pelvic and belly area, chest, shoulders, neck, head, mouth, eyes, and entire face.

- Mentally scan your body. If you find any place that's still tense, relax it and let it sink into the bed.

- Allow yourself to drift into sleep when the body and mind are ready.

Deep Breathing (particularly effective when done after Progressive Relaxation)

One of the main reasons many of us are tense is our breathing. Most people breathe very shallowly, using only the top part of their lungs. Deep Breathing allows us to use our entire lungs, providing more oxygen to our bodies and energizing and rejuvenating every organ and cell in our bodies. It is probably the most effective and beneficial method of relaxation we've seen.

- Lie on your back.

- Slowly relax your body, starting with your feet and moving through every part of your body until you have reached—and relaxed—your face and scalp.

- Do a quick check to see if you've missed any place. If so, relax it.

- Slowly begin to inhale; first filling your lower belly, then your stomach area, and then your chest, and the top of your lungs almost up to your shoulders. Hold for a second or two, and then begin to exhale. Empty the very bottom of your lungs first, then the middle, and finally the top.

- Continue this relaxed, peaceful breathing for four or five minutes.

- After a while, imagine that you are resting on a warm, gentle ocean. The sun is shining peacefully on your body. Imagine that you rise on the gentle swells of the water as you inhale, and that you slowly descend as you exhale.

- Continue this relaxing breathing, as the mind begins to drift, sleep will naturally follow.

Natural Sleep Aids

Some natural substances, such as herbs, promote relaxation and sleep. These natural substances may eventually lose their effectiveness over time. Use them as a last resort and only sparingly.

- **Valerian** (*Valeriana officinalis*) is an age-old herbal sleep aid. Research has shown that it not only helps you fall asleep faster but also improves the quality of your sleep. However, for a small percentage of people, it produces a stimulating rather than a sedative effect. It puts you to sleep but doesn't cause a groggy feeling in the morning. It is typically taken thirty to forty-five minutes before bedtime. It is available in capsules or in a tincture. Since products vary, follow the label instructions.

- **Kava Kava** (*Piper methysticum*) is an herb that is known to induce relaxation and natural sleep. It is typically taken one hour before bedtime. It is available in capsules or in a tincture. Since products vary, follow the label instructions.

- **Chamomile** (*Matricaria recutita*) is other age-old herbal remedy for calming nerves and promoting sleep. It is available as a tea or a tincture. The typical dosage is one to two cups of tea before bedtime.

- **Catnip** (*Nepeta cataria*) is an herb that has a gentle sedative effect. It is available as a tea. The typical dosage is one cup of tea before bedtime.

- **Melatonin** is a sleep-inducing hormone naturally produced in the brain. Production of this hormone usually begins to drop after the age of forty. Melatonin helps regulate the body's clock or sleep/wake cycle. The secretion of melatonin is increased by darkness and decreased by light. Not all medical experts agree on the safety of taking this hormone as a sleep aid and caution against taking it. The typical dose ranges between 0.5 to 3 mg taken a half-hour to an hour before bedtime.

Emotional Health

Enjoying the benefits of a healthy lifestyle encompasses not only nutrition and physical fitness, but also psychological, spiritual, social, and vocational aspects of your life. All these lifestyle behaviors have significant influence on your health, quality of life, and well-being. Making lifestyle changes takes time. It takes about three weeks for a new behavior to become a normal part of your daily life. Health experts recommend that you make only one lifestyle change at a time.

Psychological well-being combines your emotional and mental states. These change day to day. No one has total control over his or her emotional states, be it joy, sadness, fear, anger, shyness, or loneliness. Striving to maintain an emotion balance and knowing when to express emotions appropriately and comfortably is healthful. If you have mental well-being, you will have a better change of experiencing reality positively and reacting to challenges productively. You will use healthful skills to deal with stress and personal problems.

Spiritual well-being is a positive sense of whatever provides meaning, and purpose in your life. We all seek meaning to our lives. You can use your religion, beliefs, values, faith, creed, principles, morals, or ethics to describe that meaning. Knowing your purpose in life enables you to be more comfortable expressing love, joy, peace, and a sense of fulfillment. It also gives you hope, helping you endure setbacks in personal goals and unexpected turns of events so common in life. Spiritual well-being fosters a feeling of being connected with your inner self, significant others, and the universe.

Social well-being means having satisfying, trusting relationships and interacting well with other people. It means having a network of family, friends, and others who can be called upon during times of need. It gives you a sense of fairness, justice, and concern and appreciation for the diversity of people in the world.

Vocational well-being is finding meaning in and satisfaction in what you do for a living, pursing an education, and how you spend your leisure time. We need to ask ourselves if what we are doing presently in our lives is stimulating, challenging, and rewarding. If it is, we must congratulate ourselves! We are living a vital, balanced, and enriched life! If it is not, we must dig deep within ourselves and question if we should make a change and seek further training in an area of personal interest. This may lead to a change in jobs, education, or personal outlook on life in general.

When making lifestyle changes, strive for balance, engage in variety, and practice moderation. Balance indulgent behavior with ascetic behavior. Vary your daily routines, be they physical activities or the foods you eat. Variety is truly the spice of life; there is so much to experience! But experience with moderation, too much of a good thing can lead to fatigue, weight gain, and poor health. You can keep life exciting without unnecessary health risks.

Add Humor to Your Life

Humor is intended to make people laugh and feel happy. The origins of the word "humour" lie in the humoral medicine of the ancient Greeks, which stated that a mix of fluids, or humours, controlled human health and emotion. Today we have a better understanding of how laughter affects human physiology. Humor has been determined as a great health enhancer. Humor can help with the following:

- **Reduce pain:** Our bodies produce pain-killing hormones called endorphins in response to laughter.

- **Strengthen immune function:** A good belly laugh increases production of T-cells, interferon, and immune proteins called globulins.

- **Decrease stress:** When under stress, we produce a hormone called cortisol. Laughter significantly lowers cortisol levels and returns the body to a more relaxed state.

- **Have a positive impact on intellectual and emotional functioning:** It helps put life's trials and tribulations into healthy perspective by making them seem smaller. It helps us in overcoming fear, it allows us to take ourselves less seriously, and it triggers our creativity.

Joke telling, playfulness, and silliness are not just for children. A healthy dose of daily humor and laughter can add joy and playfulness to daily living. Here are a few types of humor:

- Slapstick

- Satire

- Irony

- Plays on words such as oxymorons and puns

- Wit, as in many one-liners

- Non-sequiturs

- Sarcasm

- Ridiculous gestures and movements

- Faking stupidity and pointing out real stupidity

- Silly acts inappropriate for the situation or age of person

- Playing a practical joke: Deliberately luring someone into a humorous position and then laughing at their expense

- Adages, often in the form of parodying "laws" of nature

- Unexpected outcome, such as a witty or surprise punchline

- Absurdity

- Self-inflicted embarrassing situations, such as losing one's swimming trunks after a dive

- Comic sounds or inherently funny words with certain sounds that make them amusing in a particular language

- Unintentional humor, making people laugh without trying

If you let some laughter into your life, you are likely to enjoy each day to its fullest. Find one of the following methods that works for you:

- **Go to a comedy club, watch comedies, read joke books.** Find the style of humor that you like, make it a daily part of your life, and have fun.

- **Bring humor to your work environment.** Bring kids' toys to work and keep them within reach. When you are stressed, take out a toy and play. That irate customer on the phone will have no idea that you are keeping your cool by playing with a Slinky. Place funny pictures of friends and loved ones around your office, including ones of you when you were a ridiculous-looking kid.

- **Create a humor file.** Fill it with funny cartoons, sayings, and jokes, as you run across them. When things are looking particularly grim, refer to your file. You'll get a good laugh and be able to put things back in perspective in no time.

- **Create comedy situations.** When you find yourself in a nerve-wracking situation (such as locking your keys in the car), think of how your favorite comedians would handle it.

- **For recreation, do some of the things you did as a kid.** Go to the zoo or to an amusement park; go bowling or swing on a swing set. You'll find that these activities take you away from all of your stressful thoughts. And the escape will do wonders for your attitude.

- **Exaggerate a stressful situation.** Take your situation and make it even bigger than it is. You might think this will cause more stress; however, blowing the problem up will allow you to see the absurdity of it, and afford you a great belly laugh.

7

Leading a Healthy Lifestyle for the Rest of Your Life

You now know the basics of building a healthy lifestyle. Make the most out of the rest of your life by eating well, being fit, and being at ease. Follow this simple advice throughout your life to maintain the health benefits for the long-term. You are well on your way to achieving a healthier lifestyle, preventing disease, improving your quality of life, and reducing healthcare costs.

Here are some long-term benefits of eating well, being fit, and managing stress, and how to develop your own lifelong healthy lifestyle plan.

Eat Well!

There are numerous benefits of a healthy diet and proper nutrition, such as:

- Higher energy levels
- Maintaining your weight and your body's store of nutrients
- Increased mental alertness
- Resistance to infection, illness, and disease
- A more robust immune system
- Faster healing and recuperation after an illness or injury
- Better medication effectiveness

- Better management of chronic health problems

- Increased sense of well-being

Maintaining a nutritious diet throughout your life may be hard because of the prevalence of fast food, high-fat snacks, and huge portion sizes (especially when eating out!). By following the eating plan from Chapter 4, you *can* create and maintain a long-range plan for improved eating.

- Plan your meals weekly. Plan meals at home as well as meals out.

- Know your portion sizes! Read the Nutrition Facts labels on food products. Use the food serving size determination method that works best for you: comparison, pre-measured, or hand.

- Develop your meals using the plan in Chapter 4's section, "Selecting Nourishing Foods." The building blocks of your meals should include protein, grains, vegetables and fruits, a bit of fat, and water.

- Build your breakfast, lunch, and dinner meals based on the suggestions in the Chapter 4's "Building Meals" section, and then get creative! Keep in mind the food preparation tips that are given in Appendix B. Expand your meal creations by reviewing any one of the many cookbooks featuring healthful living meal plans. Many of these meals can be prepared in thirty minutes or less! Add one new, nutritious food each week.

- If you don't have thirty minutes to prepare a meal and you are eating out, don't worry! You can make healthful food choices when dining out or eating on-the-go. Your restaurant choices may be buffets, Italian, Chinese, Mexican, fast food, or a pizza parlor. Or you may be eating at an airport, in your car, or between meetings at work. Use the healthful dining out food selections suggested in the Chapter 4's section "Eating Out."

- Even though you are eating a variety of nutritious foods, perhaps 80 percent of the time, there will be times when you succumb to less nutritious foods, so include a multivitamin and mineral supplement to make sure your daily dietary nutrient intakes are met.

- Make sure to practice good dental health daily.

Be Fit!

The long-term benefits of regular physical activity include:

- Promoting the loss of body fat by building or preserving muscle mass and improving the body's ability to use calories

- Limiting appetite

- Reducing the likelihood of regaining lost weight

- Preventing the fall in basal metabolic rate (rate at which our bodies burn calories) that we experience during a weight reduction program and that occurs with aging

- Helping process your food, allowing you a high-enough calorie intake to ensure proper nutrition without putting on extra weight

- Improving your heart health, lowering your blood pressure, raising your good cholesterol levels, and reducing your bad cholesterol levels

- Promoting bone formation and preventing many forms of bone loss associated with aging

- Preventing injury by increasing muscle strength and endurance, and improving flexibility and posture

- Improving your mood, reducing depression and anxiety, and helping you manage stress better

Maintaining physical fitness throughout your life may be hard because of demands on your time. By following the fitness plan from Chapter 5, you *can* create and maintain a long-range plan for improving and maintaining your body fitness.

- Develop an overall body fitness plan that works into your lifestyle using the suggestions given. Make sure to include the core components of fitness: flexibility, aerobics, and strengthening fitness activities.

- Find the physical activities that you like and can fit into your daily routine. The chart, Fitness Activities and Calories Burned, will help you choose new activities to prevent exercise boredom. Or incorporate the flexibility and strengthening exercises in Appendix A.

- Remember, an easy way to improve and maintain your body fitness is to add more walking in your daily routine. For example, add 10 minutes of extra brisk walking your first week, then add another 5 to 10 minutes each subsequent week to reach a 30- to 40-minute daily aerobic fitness activity. You can maintain lifetime fitness with just a walking program. So easy!

- Nurture your fit body from the outside by caring for your skin daily.

At Ease!

Just as important as good nutrition and physical fitness, managing stress throughout your life may be hard because of the nature of our societal demands. The long-term benefits of relaxation include:

- Reducing stress
- Lowering blood pressure
- Elevating mood
- Combating fatigue
- Promoting sleep
- Easing muscle tension
- Reducing pain-related stress
- Decreasing mental worries
- Increasing concentration
- Increasing clear thinking
- Increasing productivity

By following the relaxation techniques from Chapter 6, you *can* create and maintain a long-range plan for managing the daily stress in your life and improving your sleep and emotional health.

- Choose and practice daily the relaxation technique that works best for you from the techniques outlined.

- You may be sleeping better because of your improved nutrition and fitness. However, on those nights where sleep is not restful or forthcoming, sleep better by using any one of the nutritional, environmental, lifestyle, or relaxation techniques suggested.

- Review and consider the psychological, spiritual, social, and vocational aspects of your life regularly. These change throughout our lives and affect our overall emotional health. Take the time to revisit each one of these aspects at intervals during your life, whether yearly, every five years, or at a decade milestone. When you decide to make a change, keep in mind that lifestyle changes take time, so be patient and stick with it.

- Enjoy each day to its fullest with a daily dose of humor!

Congratulations! You are on your way to building a healthier lifestyle day by day. With these simple nutrition and fitness guidelines, eating well and being physically active for a lifetime may not be as hard as you think. A healthy lifestyle requires a long-term commitment, but the benefits are well worth it. And don't worry if you fall back into old eating and fitness habits, it's easy to slip back into familiar and comfortable ways. Revisit this book to get back on track again. Your body is wonderfully resilient, replenish it with good nutrition, fitness, and stress management and you will reap the rewards of lifelong good health.

Enjoy each day!

Appendix A

Flexibility and Strengthening Fitness Exercises

Flexibility

Flexibility fitness should be performed before and after Aerobic Fitness or Strength Fitness during the week. Plan on doing some type of fitness activity five to six times a week.

Keep in mind to go slowly and gently with deliberate movements, no bouncing; this is the key to creating and maintaining flexibility in your body.

Pelvic Tilt: Lie on your back with knees bent and arms at your side. Tighten stomach muscles and flatten the small of your back against the floor, without pushing down on the legs. Hold the tilt for five seconds, and then slowly relax. Repeat ten times.

Single Knee to Chest: Lie on your back with knees bent. Perform a pelvic tilt; then grasp your right knee with your hands, and gently pull your knee toward your chest. Hold for a count of 10. Return to starting position. Repeat with left leg. Do two times for each leg.

Double Knee to Chest: Lie on your back with knees bent. Perform a pelvic tilt; then grasp both knees with your hands, and gently pull toward your chest. Hold for a count of 10. Return to starting position. Do two times.

Back Rotation: Lie on your back with your right knee bent. Grasp your right knee with your left hand and gently pull to the left side until you feel a stretch. Keep your shoulders on the floor. Hold for a count of 10. Return to the starting position and repeat with your left knee. Do two times.

Hamstring Stretch: Lying on your back, grasp the back of the thigh of your right leg with both hands. Bend your hip up so your knee is facing the ceiling. Straighten your leg, raising your foot toward the ceiling. Your opposite leg should be flat against the floor. Hold for a count of 10. Return to the starting position and repeat with your left thigh. Do two times for each leg.

Heel Stretch: Lean against a wall and put your right foot forward. Keep your left foot flat and knee straight. Lower your body toward the wall by bending your elbows. Hold for a count of 10. Return to the starting position and repeat with your left leg forward and right leg stretched behind. Do two times for each leg.

Quadriceps Stretch: Brace yourself against a wall and grasp your right foot or ankle behind you. Gently pull it toward your buttocks, keeping your back straight—no arching. Hold for a count of 10. Return to the starting position and repeat with the left foot. Do two times for each leg.

Lunge: Take a large step forward with your right foot. Place your hands on your right knee and lean forward, bending your knee at a 90-degree angle, keeping your left knee in line with your left ankle. Hold for a count of 10. Return to the starting position and repeat with the left foot. Do two times for each leg.

Back Arm Stretch: With arms extended behind your back, interlace your fingers and push your arms up and back. Keep your chest out and head erect. Hold for a count of 10. Do two times.

Waist Stretch: Stand straight with your feet spread comfortably apart. Clasp your hands above your head and lean to the right from the waist. Straighten up and slowly bend to the left. Straighten up and slowly bend to the right. Bend from right to left, then left to right, two times.

Strengthening

Strength fitness should be performed two to three times a week, alternating with your Aerobic Fitness day.

When you lift weights, perform each movement slowly and deliberately. Specific weight-lifting movements are performed for a specific number of repetitions and a series of repetitions is called a set. Use 2-pound dumbbell and 1- to 1½-pound ankle weights to begin, progressing to 3- or 5-pound dumbbell, and 2½- to 5-pound ankle weights as your strength improves.

Complete the strength fitness program with the flexibility fitness program to cool down your muscles and help prevent aches and pains.

Biceps Curl: Stand straight with arms at your sides, holding a dumbbell in each hand. Bend your arms and slowly raise the dumbbell toward your shoulders. Return to the starting position by lowering the weights slowly to your sides. Do two to three sets of 8 repetitions, resting about thirty seconds between sets.

Overhead Press: Stand with your feet shoulder-width apart, holding a dumbbell in each hand. Keep your back straight and raise your hands to your shoulder. Then raise both your arms toward the ceiling, so that the weights are above your head and the end of each weight is touching the other. Return to starting position by lowering the weights slowly to shoulder level. Do two to three sets of 8 repetitions, resting about thirty seconds between sets.

French Press: Stand straight and grasp a dumbbell at one end with both hands. Lift the weight overhead, fully extending both arms. Lower the weight slowly behind your head as far as you can, keeping your elbows pointed upward. Then, return to the starting position by slowly raising the weight so your arms are fully extended. Do two to three sets of 8 repetitions, resting about thirty seconds between sets.

Lateral Raise: Stand with your feet shoulder-width apart, holding a dumbbell in each hand, with your arms at your sides. Gently raise your arms out to the sides until your elbows are slightly higher than your shoulders. Lower your arms to the starting position. Do two to three sets of 8 repetitions, resting about thirty seconds between sets.

Arm Row: Stand in front of a chair and hold a weight in your left hand. Bending at your hips, lean forward and balance yourself on the chair with your right hand. Lift the weight to your side, and gently pull your left arm up, bending your elbow, to your chest. Then bend your elbow up behind you. Return to the starting position by slowly lowering the weight. Do two to three sets of 8 repetitions, resting about thirty seconds between sets. Repeat with your right arm.

Triceps Kickback: Stand in front of a chair and hold a weight in your left hand. Bending at your hips, lean forward and balance yourself on the chair with your right hand. Lift the weight to your side, and then bend your elbow up behind you. Slowly swing your forearm back, straightening your elbow. The weight should be a just a bit above the level of your back. Return to the starting position by lowering the weight slowly. Do two to three sets of 8 repetitions, resting about thirty seconds between sets. Repeat with your right arm.

Butterfly Curl: Lie on your back on a small rug on the floor, holding a dumbbell in each hand. Extend arms to hold the weights straight above your chest. Slowly swing your hands out and lower them to the floor. Return to starting position by slowly raising the weights to above your chest. Do two to three sets of 8 repetitions, resting about thirty seconds between sets.

Push-Up: Kneeling on a small rug, lean forward and place your hands shoulder-width apart on the rug. Point your fingers inward and your elbows outward. In this upright position, your arms and back should be straight, with knees touching the floor. Slowly lower your chest to the floor, keeping your back straight. Push up slowly, straightening your arms. Return to the starting position by slowly pushing up, straightening your arms. Do two to three sets of 8 repetitions, resting about thirty seconds between sets.

Crunch Combo: Lie on your back on a small rug on the floor, with your arms across your chest or hands behind your head. Keeping your lower back on the floor, contract your abdominals and lift your shoulders. Twist your body slightly to the left and lower yourself to the floor, and then crunch forward by lifting your shoulders with no twisting. Lower, then lift and twist toward the right. Lower body and crunch forward. Return to starting position. Do two to three sets of 8 repetitions, resting about thirty seconds between sets.

Squat: Stand with your feet shoulder-width apart and your toes pointed straight ahead. With your feet flat on the floor, lower yourself into the squat position (just like sitting in a chair), extending your arms straight ahead as you do, looking forward. Keep your knees and ankles aligned; your knees should not extend beyond the ankles. Return to the starting position by slowly rising to the standing position. Do two to three sets of 8 repetitions, resting about thirty seconds between sets.

Leg Curl: Put an ankle-weight on each ankle. Holding on to the back of a chair, slowly bend your right knee until it is approximately parallel to the floor. Return to the starting position by lowering your leg slowly to the floor. Do two to three sets of 8 repetitions, resting about thirty seconds between sets. Repeat with your left leg.

Leg Lifts: With an ankle-weight on each ankle and holding onto the back of a chair, slowly lift your right leg behind you. Without straining, bending your knee slightly. Return to the starting position by slowly lowering your leg to the floor. Do two to three sets of 8 repetitions, resting about thirty seconds between sets. Repeat with your left leg.

Leg Extension: With an ankle-weight on each ankle, sit in a chair and slowly raise your right foot until your knee is straight and your leg is approximately parallel to the floor. Hold for a count of 3. Return to the starting position by slowly lowering your leg to the floor. Do two to three sets of 8 repetitions, resting about thirty seconds between sets. Repeat with your left leg

Cross Ankle Lift: With an ankle-weight on each ankle, sit in a chair and stretch out your legs in front of you. Cross your legs at the ankle and hold for a count of three. Return to the starting position by slowly lowering your leg to the floor. Do two to three sets of 8 repetitions, resting about thirty seconds between sets.

Appendix B

Food Preparation Tips

Food Safety

To insure the safety of your food supply, follow these four simple steps: clean, separate, cook, and chill.

- **Clean:** Wash your hands carefully with hot soapy water before handling food. Wash all utensils and cooking surfaces. Wash dishes, utensils, cutting boards (use non-porous types only), and countertops with hot soapy water after preparing each food.

- **Separate:** Don't cross-contaminate raw foods. Separate raw meat, poultry, fish, and eggs from all other foods in your shopping cart, in your refrigerator, and in your freezer. Don't cross-contaminate in cooking. While cooking, use one cutting board for raw meats and another for produce and ready-to-eat foods.

- **Cook:** Prepare all foods at proper temperatures. All foods must be cooked long enough and at a high enough temperature to kill bacteria that cause food-borne illnesses. Use a food thermometer rather than the color of the food, to judge if it has reached the proper internal temperature. Cook steaks and roasts to 145° F, ground beef to 160° F, and chicken breasts to 170° F. In terms of food safety, slightly overcooked is always better than underdone.

- **Chill:** Refrigerate raw foods and leftovers promptly. Refrigerate perishable foods, prepared food, and all leftovers within two hours. Defrost and marinate all foods in the fridge. Never defrost foods at room temperature or marinate meats outside of the refrigerator. Thaw frozen food in the fridge, in a microwave, or under cold running water in the sink. Marinate meat, poultry, and fish inside the refrigerator in a leak-proof plastic bag or covered container.

When your mother said, "If in doubt, throw it out," she was right again. If food has been left out for too long or refrigerated for too long, it may not be safe to eat even if it looks and smells fine.

Preparing Greens

Greens, such as collards, kales, chard, beet, or mustard greens, have strong tastes. Beet greens and chard contain oxalic acid giving the vegetables a sharp, somewhat bitter flavor. Ill-prepared (overcooked) greens usually have an olive drab color, stringy texture, and unappetizing flavor. Gently sautéing greens just until they wilt will give them a bright green color and succulent texture. A good mix is one part greens to approximately two parts spinach, which tempers the strong flavor of that particular green. Removing the tough central stalks will also eliminate any stringiness during cooking. In general, follow these steps when preparing greens:

- Wash them gently in mild dish detergent to remove any dirt and lingering pesticides. Rinse in warm water and drain in a colander.

- On a cutting board, remove the tough central stalks, stems, and midribs by placing the leaf facedown on the board and cutting out the stalk, leaving the leaf in a V-shape. Once all the leaves have been trimmed, stack them up and cut the leaves into shreds.

- Chop ½ large onion and mince 2 or 3 cloves of garlic (or use 1 teaspoon of prepared minced garlic).

- In a large skillet or Dutch oven, heat 2 tablespoons of extra-virgin olive oil.

- Add the onions, sautéing over medium heat until just tender, stir in the greens a bit at a time, tossing it about as it wilts.

- When all the greens have been added and are slightly wilted (they will have a vivid green color), stir in the garlic, mixing it well among the greens. Sauté for no more than a minute.

- Season with salt and pepper to taste and serve immediately.

Preparing Broccoli and the Cabbage Family

Broccoli is one of the healthiest members of crucifers or cabbage family. These types of vegetables have significant anticancer properties, as well as fiber. As with the greens, ill-prepared broccoli, Brussels sprouts, and green cabbage can have that odoriferous sulfur smell and taste and olive drab color. To maintain the bright color of these vegetables, cook them gently in a small amount of water or gently sauté them. Once you've cooked these vegetables using these methods, you'll want them more than once a week!

To cook broccoli, cauliflower, and Brussels sprouts, without sautéing:

- Wash gently in mild dish detergent to remove any dirt and lingering pesticides. Rinse in warm water. Drain in a colander.

- Cut the end of the woody stem off the broccoli or cauliflower stalk. Cut the remaining stalk off just below the florets. Cut the stem pieces into bite-size pieces. Separate each floret.

- Mince 1 or 2 cloves of garlic or use 1 teaspoon of prepared minced garlic.

- In a heavy saucepan, heat a small amount of water to just a boil. Place broccoli, cauliflower, or Brussels sprouts in the water. Add 1 tablespoon of extra-virgin olive oil. Cover and lower the heat. Add the garlic after about a minute. Cook until the vegetables are crisp-tender.

Sautéing cabbage:

- Wash gently in mild dish detergent to remove any dirt and lingering pesticides. Rinse in warm water. Drain in a colander.

- On a cutting board, remove the tough central stalks, stems, and midribs by placing the leaf facedown on the board and cutting out the stalk, leaving the leaf in a V-shape. Once all the leaves have been trimmed, stack them up and cut the leaves into shreds.

- Mince 2 or 3 cloves of garlic (or use 1 teaspoon of prepared minced garlic).

- In a large skillet or Dutch oven, heat 2 tablespoons of extra-virgin olive oil.

- Stir in the cabbage a bit at a time, sautéing until just crisp-tender. Add the garlic and cook for no more than a minute.

- Season with salt and pepper to taste and serve immediately.

APPENDIX C

Resources

Books and Audiocassettes

Atkins, Robert, M.D. *Dr. Atkins' Age-Defying Diet*. New York: St. Martin's Press, 2001.

Atkins, Robert, M.D. *Dr. Atkins' New Diet Revolution*. New York: Harper-Collins, 2002.

Benson, Herbert, M.D. *The Relaxation Response*. New York: HarperTorch, 2000.

Borushek, Allan. *The Doctor's Pocket Calorie, Fat and Carbohydrate Counter*. Costa Mesa, CA: Family Health Publications, 2003.

Cousins, Norman. *Anatomy of an Illness*. New York: Bantam, 1981.

Editors of Prevention Magazine Health Books. *The Female Body: An Owner's Manual*. Rodale Press, 1996.

Jacobson, Michael, Ph.D. and Hurley, Janyne, Ph.D. *Restaurant Confidential*. New York: Workman Publishing Company, Inc., 2002.

Kabat-Zinn, Jon. *Wherever You Go, There You Are: Mindfulness Meditation in Everyday Life*. New York: Hyperion, 1994.

Northrup, Christiane, M.D. *The Wisdom of Menopause: Creating Physical and Emotional Health and Healing During the Change.* New York: Bantam Books, 2001.

Perrione, Nicholas, M.D. *The Perricone Prescription.* New York: HarperCollins, 2002.

Siegel, Bernie, M.D. *Humor and Healing.* Audiocassette. Sounds True, 1997.

Sutcliffe, Jenny. *The Complete Book of Relaxation Techniques.* Allentown, PA: People's Medical Society, 1994.

Weil, Andrew, M.D. *Natural Health, Natural Medicine.* New York: Houghton Mifflin, 1995.

Weil, Andrew, M.D. *Eight Weeks to Optimum Health.* New York: Ballantine Books, 1997.

Weil, Andrew, M.D. *Eating for Optimum Health.* New York: Alfred A. Knopf, 2000.

Whitaker, Julian, M.D., and Colman, Carol. *Shed Ten Years in Ten Weeks.* New York: Simon and Schuster, 1997.

Web Sites

ConsumerLab.com, LLC, provides independent test results and information to help consumers and health care professionals evaluate health, wellness, and nutrition products. It publishes results of its tests online information to help consumers and health care professionals evaluate health, wellness, and nutrition products, www.ConsumerLab.com

FDA Center for Food Safety and Applied Nutrition, U.S. Department of Health and Human Services, US Environmental Protection Agency. www.cfsan.fda.gov

FDA Guide to Dietary Supplements. www.fda.gov

Filtered Water Pitcher Systems. www.brita.com, www.purwater.com

Glycemic Index of Foods. www.joslin.harvard.edu/educate/library/glycemic_index.shtml, www.healthcheckssytems.com/glycemic.htm

Health and fitness. www.cdc.gov, www.pueblo.gsa.gov

Healthfinder, Your Guide to Reliable Health Information. www.healthfinder.gov

Information on herbs, vitamins, and dietary supplements. www.rxmed.com and www.herbs2000.com American Botanical Council, common herbs, herb reference guide. www.herbalgram.org.

Information on skin care and products in general. www.smartskincare.com

Institute of Medicine of the National Academies. www.iom.edu

International Food Information Council. www.ific.org

Stress Management. www.stress.about.com

USDA 2000 Dietary Guidelines for Americans. www.health.gov

USDA Food and Nutrition Information Center, USDA Nutrient Data Laboratory. www.nal.usda.gov

About the Author

Mary El-Baz has a B.S. and a M.S. from the University of Missouri and is the author of several business and technical publications. She is an Herbal Information Specialist and a Pharmacy Technician. Her main focus is the body and mind benefits of nutritious foods. She has enjoyed good nutrition and fitness throughout the years, from general nutritional advice and its affect on one's overall health from Adelle Davis, to the advice of natural and preventive medicine specialists discussing the more recent scientific findings on how the nutrients in our foods create and maintain our health. She is currently pursuing a Doctor of Philosophy in Holistic Nutrition.

Index

0-595-32506-8

www.ingramcontent.com/pod-product-compliance
Lightning Source LLC
Chambersburg PA
CBHW020251290526
45784CB00003B/1195